T0259547

Foot and Ankle Arthrodesis

Editor

JOHN J. STAPLETON

CLINICS IN PODIATRIC MEDICINE AND SURGERY

www.podiatric.theclinics.com

Consulting Editor
THOMAS ZGONIS

July 2017 • Volume 34 • Number 3

ELSEVIER

1600 John F. Kennedy Boulevard • Suite 1800 • Philadelphia, Pennsylvania, 19103-2899

http://www.theclinics.com

CLINICS IN PODIATRIC MEDICINE AND SURGERY Volume 34, Number 3
July 2017 ISSN 0891-8422, ISBN-13: 978-0-323-53150-4

Editor: Lauren Boyle
Developmental Editor: Alison Swety

Clinics in Podiatric Medicine and Surgery (ISSN 0891-8422) is published quarterly by Elsevier Inc., 360 Park Avenue South, New York, NY 10010-1710. Months of issue are January, April, July, and October. Business and Editorial Offices: 1600 John F. Kennedy Blvd., Ste. 1800, Philadelphia, PA 19103-2899. Customer Service Office: 3251 Riverport Lane, Maryland Heights, MO 63043. Periodicals postage paid at New York, NY and additional mailing offices. Subscription prices are $288.00 per year for US individuals, $518.00 per year for US institutions, $100.00 per year for US students and residents, $374.00 per year for Canadian individuals, $626.00 for Canadian institutions, $439.00 for international individuals, $626.00 per year for international institutions and $220.00 per year for Canadian and foreign students/residents. To receive student/resident rate, orders must be accompanied by name of affiliated institution, date of term, and the *signature* of program/residency coordinator on institution letterhead. Orders will be billed at individual rate until proof of status is received. Foreign air speed delivery is included in all *Clinics* subscription prices. All prices are subject to change without notice. POSTMASTER: Send address changes to *Clinics in Podiatric Medicine and Surgery*, Elsevier Health Sciences Division, Subscription Customer Service, 3251 Riverport Lane, Maryland Heights, MO 63043. **Customer Service: 1-800-654-2452 (US). From outside of the US, call 314-447-8871. Fax: 314-447-8029. E-mail: JournalsCustomerService-usa@elsevier.com (for print support); JournalsOnlineSupport-usa@elsevier.com (for online support).**

Reprints. For copies of 100 or more of articles in this publication, please contact the Commercial Reprints Department, Elsevier Inc., 360 Park Avenue South, New York, NY 10010-1710. Tel.: 212-633-3874; Fax: 212-633-3820; E-mail: reprints@elsevier.com.

Clinics in Podiatric Medicine and Surgery is covered in *MEDLINE/PubMed (Index Medicus)* and *EMBASE/Excerpta Medica.*

CLINICS IN PODIATRIC MEDICINE AND SURGERY

Contributors

CONSULTING EDITOR

THOMAS ZGONIS, DPM, FACFAS
Professor and Director, Externship and Reconstructive Foot and Ankle Surgery Fellowship Programs, Division of Podiatric Medicine and Surgery, Department of Orthopaedics, University of Texas Health Science Center San Antonio, San Antonio, Texas

EDITOR

JOHN J. STAPLETON, DPM, FACFAS
Foot and Ankle Surgery, LVPG Orthopaedics and Chief of Podiatric Surgery, Lehigh Valley Hospital, Allentown, Pennsylvania; Clinical Assistant Professor of Surgery, Penn State College of Medicine, Hershey, Pennsylvania

AUTHORS

NICHOLAS J. BEVILACQUA, DPM, FACFAS
Associate, Foot and Ankle Surgery, North Jersey Orthopaedic Specialists, Teaneck, New Jersey

PATRICK R. BURNS, DPM
Podiatric Medicine and Surgery Residency, Department of Orthopaedic Surgery, Director, University of Pittsburgh Medical Center, Assistant Professor, University of Pittsburgh School of Medicine, Pittsburgh, Pennsylvania

DANIELLE N. BUTTO, DPM, AACFAS
St. Francis Hospital and Medical Center, Hartford, Connecticut

CATHERINE L. CHURCHILL, DPM
Attending Physician, Department of Podiatric Surgery, Jersey Shore University Medical Center, Neptune, New Jersey

LAWRENCE A. DiDOMENICO, DPM, FACFAS
Director of Residency Training, Northside Hospital; Director of Fellowship Training, Ankle and Foot Care Centers, KSU College of Podiatric Medicine; Section Chief of Podiatric Medicine and Surgery, St. Elizabeth Hospital, Youngstown, Ohio

AUGUSTA DUNSE, DPM
PGY-2, Podiatric Medicine and Surgery Residency, University of Pittsburgh Medical Center, Pittsburgh, Pennsylvania

GEOFFREY G. HALLOCK, MD
Division of Plastic Surgery, Sacred Heart Hospital, The Lehigh Valley Hospital, Allentown, Pennsylvania

CRYSTAL L. RAMANUJAM, DPM, MSc
Assistant Professor/Clinical, Division of Podiatric Medicine and Surgery, Department of Orthopaedics, University of Texas Health Science Center San Antonio, San Antonio, Texas

THOMAS S. ROUKIS, DPM, PhD, FACFAS
Past President, American College of Foot and Ankle Surgeons, Department of Orthopaedics, Podiatry and Sports Medicine, Orthopaedic Center, Gundersen Health System, La Crosse, Wisconsin

DANIEL J. SHORT, DPM
Attending Faculty, Mid-Atlantic Permanente Medical Group, Springfield Medical Center, Springfield, Virginia

JOHN J. STAPLETON, DPM, FACFAS
Foot and Ankle Surgery, LVPG Orthopaedics and Chief of Podiatric Surgery, Lehigh Valley Hospital, Allentown, Pennsylvania; Clinical Assistant Professor of Surgery, Penn State College of Medicine, Hershey, Pennsylvania

JAMES P. SULLIVAN, DPM
Podiatric Surgery Residency Director, Department of Podiatric Surgery, Jersey Shore University Medical Center, Neptune, New Jersey

GEORGE F. WALLACE, DPM, MBA
Director, Podiatry Service, Medical Director, Ambulatory Care Services, University Hospital, Newark, New Jersey

THOMAS ZGONIS, DPM, FACFAS
Professor and Director, Externship and Reconstructive Foot and Ankle Surgery Fellowship Programs, Division of Podiatric Medicine and Surgery, Department of Orthopaedics, University of Texas Health Science Center San Antonio, San Antonio, Texas

Contents

patient satisfaction with low complications while preserving motion in adjacent tarsal joints. Joint preparation is important and time should be spent preparing the joint for successful arthrodesis and the fixation construct needs to be done well and effectively to provide a solid Arbeitsgemeinschaft für Osteosynthesefragen (AO) construct for good results.

Triple (talonavicular, subtalar, and calcaneocuboid) joint arthrodesis and most recently double (talonavicular and subtalar) joint arthrodesis have been well proposed in the literature for surgical repair of the elective, posttraumatic, and/or neuropathic hindfoot deformities. The articulation of the hindfoot with the ankle and midfoot is multiaxial, and arthrodesis of these joints can significantly alter the lower extremity biomechanical manifestations by providing anatomic correction and alignment. This article reviews the indications and preoperative planning for some of the most common procedures to address the hindfoot deformity.

Ankle arthrodesis remains one of the most definitive treatment options for end-stage arthritis, paralysis, posttraumatic and postinfectious conditions, failed total ankle arthroplasty, and severe deformities. The general aims of ankle arthrodesis are to decrease pain and instability, correct the accompanying deformity, and create a stable plantigrade foot. Several surgical approaches have been reported for ankle arthrodesis with internal fixation options. External fixation has also evolved for ankle arthrodesis in certain clinical scenarios. This article provides a comprehensive analysis of midterm to long-term outcomes for ankle arthrodesis using internal and/or external fixation each for elective and diabetic conditions.

Tibiotalocalcaneal arthrodesis is a safe and viable option to treat patients with arthridities affecting ankle and subtalar joints, neuromuscular disorders, avascular necrosis of the talus, failed ankle arthrodesis, instability, and Charcot neuroarthropathy. Choice of incision and fixation is based on deformity, pathology, prior surgery and hardware, and surgeon comfort and preference. Intramedullary nails offer high primary stability, reduce sustained soft tissue damage, and may allow for earlier return to activities than traditional plate or screw constructs. Peri- and postoperative fractures, malunion, nonunion, and infections are potential complications. Postoperative recovery is a vital component for an overall successful outcome.

Bone loss and destruction due to diabetic Charcot neuroarthropathy (CN) and osteomyelitis of the foot and ankle is a challenging clinical condition when lower extremity preservation is considered. Resection and excision of osteomyelitis and associated nonviable soft tissue can lead into large osseous and soft tissue defects that will most likely need the utilization of bone grafting and subsequent arthrodesis for stability and anatomic alignment. In the diabetic population with peripheral neuropathy, osseous instability can lead to subsequent lower extremity deformity, ulceration, infection and/or amputation. This article reviews the surgical approach in the presence of diabetic CN and concomitant osteomyelitis.

Unlike the traumatic "mangled" foot and ankle in which amputation could be an acceptable if not preferred option, revisional foot and ankle surgery starts with a viable foot that is then injured by the surgeon hopefully to benefit the patient. Any untoward sequela, such as inadequate wound healing, instead always requires consideration of limb salvage. Unfortunately, this may not be so simple. A proactive approach to solve this problem in a timely fashion is important. The goal must always be to get a healed wound so the final result improves the ability for independent ambulation by the patient.

A fusion rate of 100% would be ideal. Despite adhering to sound surgical principles, complete compliance, and no adverse comorbidities, that 100% fusion rate goal is elusive. Orthobiologics are a special class of materials developed to enhance the fusion rates in foot and ankle arthrodesis sites. Whether orthobiologics are used for the first fusion or reserved for a nonunion is debatable, especially when considering cost.

CLINICS IN PODIATRIC MEDICINE AND SURGERY

RELATED INTEREST

Foot and Ankle Clinics, December 2016 (Vol. 21, Issue 4)
Bone Grafts, Bone Graft Substitutes, and Biologics in Foot and Ankle Surgery
Sheldon Lin, *Editor*
Available at: http://www.foot.theclinics.com/

THE CLINICS ARE AVAILABLE ONLINE!
Access your subscription at:
www.theclinics.com

Preface

Foot and Ankle Arthrodesis

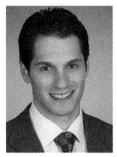

John J. Stapleton, DPM, FACFAS
Editor

Arthrodesis procedures of the foot and ankle are used to treat a variety of foot and ankle disorders. While the concept of joint arthrodesis is not new, the techniques and technological advances to perform these procedures have evolved over time. Similarly, the basic principles of soft tissue handling, meticulous joint preparation, joint alignment, stable fixation, and postoperative management are often the difference between a successful and failed arthrodesis procedure.

As guest editor, I am fortunate to have contributions from many experienced authors dealing with elective and revision foot and ankle arthrodesis procedures. The articles in this issue present multiple tips, pearls, and pitfalls to arthrodesis procedures of the foot and ankle. In addition, the role of successful free tissue transfer to manage devastating soft tissue complications arising from arthrodesis procedures is well covered for the complex postoperative cases with the need of soft tissue coverage.

Finally, I would like to thank the inviting authors for their contributions and hope that this issue will become a great reference for all readers when managing arthrodesis procedures of the foot and ankle.

John J. Stapleton, DPM, FACFAS
Foot and Ankle Surgery
LVPG Orthopaedics
Allentown, PA 18103, USA

E-mail address:
jostaple@hotmail.com

Clin Podiatr Med Surg 34 (2017) xi
http://dx.doi.org/10.1016/j.cpm.2017.04.001
0891-8422/17/© 2017 Published by Elsevier Inc.

podiatric.theclinics.com

Digital Arthrodesis of the Lesser Toes

James P. Sullivan, DPM, Catherine L. Churchill, DPM*

KEYWORDS

- Hammer toe • Digital deformities • Digital arthrodesis • Intramedullary implant

KEY POINTS

- Arthrodesis of the proximal interphalangeal joint is a popular procedure for hammer toe correction.
- Fusion of the interphalangeal joint can be fixated with a variety of methods, including K-wire fixation, intramedullary implants, absorbable pins, and screws.
- Each method of fixation has advantages and disadvantages, such as variations in complication rates, cost, and fusion rates.

INTRODUCTION

Digital deformities are commonly encountered by foot and ankle surgeons. They can be isolated deformities, or they can be associated with other forefoot, midfoot, and hindfoot pathologies. Lesser toe deformities include hammer toes, claw toes, and mallet toes. These terms have been used interchangeably, leading to some confusion with regard to nomenclature. For the purpose of this review, a hammer toe involves a flexion deformity of the proximal interphalangeal joint (PIPJ) and extension of the metatarsophalangeal joint (MTPJ). A claw toe is an extension of the MTPJ with flexion contracture of the PIPJ and distal interphalangeal joint (DIPJ), whereas a mallet toe involves a flexion contracture of the DIPJ.

The etiologies of hammer toes, claw toes, and mallet toes are debatable. Biomechanical dysfunction, however, is accepted as the main factor contributing to development of digital contractures. Shoe-gear also may play a role in the development of hammer toe deformities. Notably, lesser digital deformities and bunions are rarely seen in societies in which shoe-gear is uncommon.[1] DuVries[2] postulated that shoe-gear limits normal joint motion in the forefoot, thereby impeding the action of the intrinsic muscles of the forefoot and leading to digital contractures. These deformities

Disclosure: The authors have nothing to disclose.
Department of Podiatric Surgery, Jersey Shore University Medical Center, 1945 State Route 33, Neptune, NJ 07753, USA
* Corresponding author.
E-mail address: catherinechurchill@gmail.com

Clin Podiatr Med Surg 34 (2017) 289–300
http://dx.doi.org/10.1016/j.cpm.2017.02.001
0891-8422/17/© 2017 Elsevier Inc. All rights reserved.

can range in severity from mild, flexible deformities, to rigid, nonreducible contractures that can lead to painful digital ulcerations. Nonoperative treatments include digital strappings, shoe-gear modifications, activity modifications, and orthotics for metatarsalgia. When conservative treatment fails to alleviate pain, surgery may be warranted.

A variety of surgical procedures have been performed over the past century. Digital arthroplasty is a common procedure that may provide good short-term results, but sometimes leaves patients with inadequate correction of the digital contracture and residual deformity. Lemm and colleagues[3] demonstrated that PIPJ arthrodesis was superior to PIPJ arthroplasty in terms of toe purchase, stability, and sagittal plane correction. Other digital procedures, such as tendon transfer, tendon lengthening, and plantar plate repair, are beyond the scope of this review. Our discussion will be limited to PIPJ arthrodesis for the treatment of lesser digital deformities. With regard to PIPJ arthrodesis, a wide range of fixation techniques have been described. Fixation techniques include single or multiple Kirschner wires (K-wires),[4,5] suture,[6] intraosseous loop of stainless steel wire,[7] absorbable pin,[8] intramedullary screw,[9] and single or multicomponent metal and cortical bone allograft intramedullary implant.[10,11]

PREOPERATIVE PLANNING

When examining a patient preoperatively, it is imperative to assess the circulatory and sensory status of the patient's lower extremity. The plantar foot is evaluated for calluses and intractable plantar keratoses, which may occur secondary to retrograde buckling of the toe causing plantarflexion of the respective metatarsal head. The digit itself is evaluated for lesions, which may develop at the tip of the toe or the dorsal aspect of the PIPJ. Contractures at the MTPJ, PIPJ, and DIPJ should be carefully evaluated and documented. Medial or lateral deviation of the digit at the MTPJ level or extreme subluxation of the toe at the MTPJ level can indicate a plantar plate tear.

Lesser toe deformities may be flexible, semiflexible, or rigid. In general, the more rigid the deformity, the poorer the response to conservative treatment, necessitating an arthrodesis-type procedure. Preoperatively, the position of the digit should be evaluated in the weight-bearing position. If there is an extension contracture at the MTPJ, arthrodesis of only the PIPJ will leave the patient with a digit that elevates at the MTPJ level. MTPJ deformity also should be addressed at the time of surgery with a method such as a capsulotomy/soft tissue release. A K-wire is often placed across the MTPJ to provide the digit stability throughout the healing process. Independent single K-wire fixation across the MTPJ may also be necessary in conjunction with a metatarsal shortening procedure, such as a Weil procedure. When digital arthrodesis is being performed in conjunction with a plantar plate repair, it is often best to fixate the MTPJ temporarily, as well.

Position of the hallux also should be evaluated. If the patient has a hallux valgus deformity with a painful second toe hammertoe contracture, then there may be inadequate space between the first and third toes for the surgically corrected second toe if the concomitant bunion deformity is not also surgically addressed.

Radiographs of the foot should be performed. An anteroposterior (AP) radiograph may demonstrate diminished MTPJ joint space or even overlap of the proximal phalanx on the metatarsal head, indicating a dislocation at the MTPJ level. A "gun-barrel" sign may be visible on the AP view. If the proximal phalanx is sufficiently dislocated, it is viewed end-on, appearing as a round cylinder on the AP view of radiograph, akin to "looking down a gun barrel." Transverse plane deformities, such as medial or lateral deviations of the digit, also are visible on the AP view. A lateral radiograph is useful in determining the severity of the contracture in the sagittal plane (**Fig. 1**).

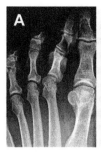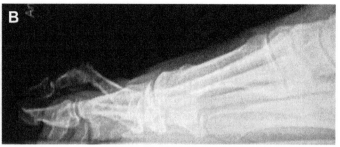

Fig. 1. (*A, B*) Lesser digit hammer toe deformities on AP and lateral radiographs.

SURGICAL TECHNIQUE

Surgery is performed with the patient in the supine position. Frequently, an ankle tourniquet is used. Some surgeons use a mixture of local anesthetic with epinephrine to obtain hemostasis in place of a tourniquet. Multiple studies demonstrate that epinephrine is safe to use in digital surgery, but should be avoided in patients with a history of arterial disease or vasculitis.[12,13]

A variety of incisional approaches have been described for the PIPJ arthrodesis. The authors' preferred incisional technique involves a dorsal longitudinal incision over the midline of the digit centered over the PIPJ. A double semi-elliptical skin wedge can be removed over the PIPJ if there is an associated skin lesion. The incision is carried proximally over the metatarsal shaft if a MTPJ release is also performed. Superficial veins are commonly encountered over the dorsal aspect of the metatarsal head and are clamped and cauterized as necessary.

The superficial fascia is then separated from the deep fascia. Neurovascular structures at the medial and lateral aspect of the incision are carefully retracted with skin hooks. Attention is directed to the proximal interphalangeal joint of the digit. The extensor tendon trifurcation is transversely transected using a 15 blade, and a PIPJ capsulotomy is performed. The medial and lateral collateral ligaments are released.

The extensor tendon is reflected proximally off the head of the proximal phalanx to expose the articular surface. The remaining distal extensor tendon is also reflected off the base of the middle phalanx to expose the articular surface. When performing an end-to-end arthrodesis, a sagittal saw or oscillating saw can be used to remove the articular cartilage from both sides of the joint. Alternatively, bone-cutting forceps can be used to remove the medial and lateral condyles, articular cartilage, and subchondral bone. Alternatively, the interphalangeal joint can be prepared for arthrodesis with a convex and concave cannulated reamer system to remove cartilage from both sides of the interphalangeal joint.

Other modifications to the digital arthrodesis technique have been described as alternatives to the end-to-end arthrodesis. A peg-in-hole arthrodesis is a more technically challenging method of arthrodesis, involving the creation of a peg at the distal end of the proximal phalanx that is then inserted into a rectangular shaped slot that has been surgically created in the base of the middle phalanx. This arthrodesis method results in more digital shortening than the traditional end-to-end arthrodesis method, but affords greater frontal plane stability.[14] There is also risk for fracture of the dorsal cortex of the proximal phalanx with this method.[15] An alternative arthrodesis technique is the "V," or "chevron," arthrodesis. This involves the surgeon creating a "V," or "herring-bone," shaped interface for arthrodesis, providing increased rotational stability in comparison with the end-to-end arthrodesis. Disadvantages of this method include digital shortening and the need for more surgical exposure of the middle phalanx for creation of the bone cuts[15] (**Fig. 2**).

After completing joint resection, the Kelikian push-up test is performed to determine if further soft tissue release is necessary to reduce the digital contracture. A Z-plasty extensor tendon lengthening is sometimes performed. A dorsal capsulotomy of the MTPJ also may be performed. If a transverse deformity is present at the MTPJ level, such as a laterally deviated digit, the lateral aspect of the MTPJ capsule is released. In some cases, the plantar plate is firmly adhered to the plantar aspect of the metatarsal head. A McGlamry elevator is used to release the plantar plate from the metatarsal head. The foot is then reloaded to determine if adequate soft tissue release has been performed. Cases of extreme subluxation or dislocation at the MTPJ level require plantar plate repair. A tenotomy of the flexor tendons also may be necessary to reduce a plantarflexion contracture at the DIPJ. This may be done from a plantar percutaneous approach or from a dorsal approach prior to fixation of the digit.

The PIPJ arthrodesis site is fixated by a variety of methods, which will be described in further detail later in this text. The extensor tendon is repaired under appropriate physiologic tension using absorbable suture. The subcutaneous tissue and skin are closed by surgeon's preference.

PIN FIXATION

Temporary single K-wire fixation has been the most common fixation method for PIPJ arthrodesis since its original description by Taylor in 1940.[4] It has been the favored fixation method by many surgeons due to the ease of insertion, minimal need for instrumentation, and maintenance of alignment.[5] Furthermore, the pin can be easily

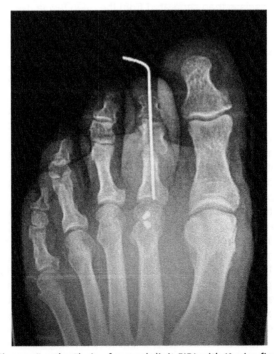

Fig. 2. "V" or "Chevron" arthrodesis of second digit PIPJ with K-wire fixation.

removed in cases of infection, malalignment, or vascular embarrassment. Traditional fixation involves antegrade insertion of a K-wire at the base of the middle phalanx through the distal aspect of the toe, followed by retrograde insertion of the wire across the PIPJ. A helpful pearl for placement and alignment of the antegrade wire is to bisect the nail plate dorsally with a skin marker. Using that bisection line as a guide is an excellent way to ensure proper alignment and placement of the K-wire in the transverse plane. The wire can be further retrograded across the MTPJ as necessary. The wire is bent at the tip and cut distally. The wire is left in place for 3 to 6 weeks and is removed in the office.

Many patients, however, have anxiety about having an external pin that must be removed at a later date. Furthermore, patients may find the pin inconveniently limits their ability to shower and to wear normal shoe-gear. Additional concerns include pin-site infections, broken fixation, and rotational instability of the digit.[5] Fixation with a single K-wire offers one point of fixation leading to rotational instability of the digit. To address rotational instability, Boffeli[5] described a 2-pin fixation method for PIPJ arthrodesis. Two parallel 0.045-inch K-wires were placed in a similar technique as the single K-wire fixation method. Boffeli's retrospective review of 91 digits treated with the 2-pin fixation method revealed a 2% complication rate. Complications included broken hardware and pin loosening, supporting the 2-pin construct as a viable fixation technique for PIPJ arthrodesis. The authors observed increased stability against rotational and bending forces with the 2-wire technique.

An additional disadvantage to K-wire fixation is the risk for pin-tract infection. Pin-tract infection rates vary in the literature. Reece and colleagues[16] reported infection rates as high as 18%, whereas Kramer and colleagues[17] reported infection rates as low as 0.3% in large review of 2698 hammer toes.[17] Other complications associated with K-wires include pin migration and breakage.[18] Zingas and colleagues[18] reported a 2.5% hardware failure rate when using 0.045 K-wires for fixation, left in for 6 weeks (**Fig. 3**).

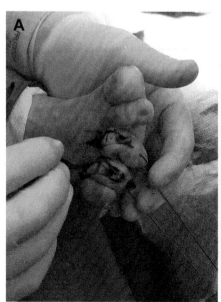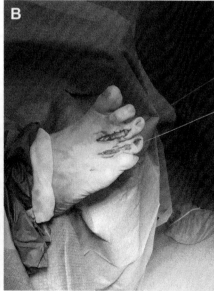

Fig. 3. (*A, B*) Single K-wire fixation in the third and fourth digits with an end-to-end arthrodesis.

ABSORBABLE INTRAMEDULLARY PINS

Absorbable pins also have been used for fixation of the PIPJ fusion site. Some absorbable pins have pointed tips and many can be placed on power instrumentation used for the insertion of standard K-wires. The pins can be trimmed at the tip of the toe so that no portion of the pin is external. Unlike K-wires, there is no routine need to remove the pin. The absorbable pin also remains in place much longer than a traditional K-wire, facilitating fusion across the arthrodesis site.

In 2007, Konkel and colleagues[8] reported on the use of poly-P-Dioxanone (PDS) absorbable pins for PIPJ fixation. They reported a 15% incidence of medial drifting of the second toe after implantation into the second PIPJ. In 2011, Konkel and colleagues[19] reported on their results using the Trim-It Drill pin (Arthrex, Inc, Naples, FL), which is made of poly L-lactate (PLLA). In this retrospective review on 47 toes, there were no hardware complications. They reported an 83% fusion rate, a 3% patient dissatisfaction rate, and no symptomatic medial or lateral digital angulation.[19] Konkel and colleagues[19] observed that using the thicker PLLA pin was preferable to the PDS pin. PLLA pins were associated with higher rates of union, less transverse and coronal plane deviation, and higher patient satisfaction rates when compared with PDS pins.

Complications with these absorbable devices include prolonged digital swelling and difficulty of hardware removal if removal becomes necessary. Marrow edema, secondary to pin resorption, is an infrequent complication, and typically resolves with time.[19] Infrequently, cystic erosion in the bone can be seen on radiographs as the pins are absorbed by hydrolysis within the body.[20] Absorbable pins are more expensive and less rigid than K-wires, making them prone to bending and breakage. Like K-wires, they do not provide rotational stability to the digit in the frontal plane, nor do they provide compression across the arthrodesis site.

IMPLANTS

In recent years, there has been an explosion of digital intramedullary implant devices on the market. Popularity of digital implants designed for PIPJ fusion has skyrocketed as new implantable devices are touted for their ability to minimize the risk of pin-tract infections and eliminate the need for external hardware. The exact surgical technique for insertion of metal hammer toe implants varies based on product design. One-piece and 2-piece designs are available. Some designs are barbed or threaded at the ends. Some devices are cannulated, allowing concomitant insertion of a K-wire across the MTPJ.

Studies regarding hammer toe implants, in general, compare implants with single K-wire fixation for PIPJ arthrodesis. Coughlin and colleagues[21] found an 81% fusion rate and 5% complication rate in a review of 118 arthrodesis procedures fixated with a single K-wire. This study followed patients over a 3-year period and excluded patients with diabetes and rheumatoid arthritis. The toe was stabilized with a single 0.045 K-wire. Infection was observed in 3 digits and malalignment in 18 of the 118 digits. The Coughlin study is commonly referenced in the intramedullary implant literature for comparison of implant devices with single K-wire fixation.

Jay and colleagues[11] reported on a randomized control trial comparing PIPJ arthrodesis with K-wire fixation to arthrodesis with a 2-component intramedullary implant. They reported no statistically significant difference between the fixation groups with regard to complication rates. However, in the implant group, they found an increased fusion rate as well as better foot-related quality-of-life outcomes. Ellington and colleagues[22] reported on a 2-piece implant used in 38 PIPJ arthrodesis procedures. The union rate for the 2-piece implant was 60.5%, with 3 hardware failures and 3 intraoperative fractures.

Witt and Hyer[10] reported a case series of 7 PIPJ arthrodesis procedures with a 1-piece intramedullary, stainless steel implant (PRO-TOE; Wright Medical Technology, Inc, Arlington, TN). No intraoperative or postoperative complications occurred during a 1-year follow-up period, and they reported the implant is a viable alternative to K-wire fixation for digital arthrodesis. They described several advantages to this particular design, including the barbed end of the implant, which is designed in a fashion to reduce rotational instability. Witt and Hyer[10] theorized that a 1-piece implant is a stronger construct than a 2-piece device, because the implant cannot uncouple, leading to a potential source of device failure.

In a retrospective review by Angirasa and colleagues,[23] the 1-piece metal SmartToe Implant (MMI USA, Inc, Memphis, TN) was compared with single K-wire fixation. Fifteen patients received single K-wire fixation, and 13 patients were fixated with the SmartToe. All patients were immobilized in a walking boot postoperatively. The patients in the K-wire group had the pin removed at 4 weeks. By 6 months, 100% of patients in the implant group had achieved radiographic fusion compared with 60% in the K-wire group. Additionally, the implant group returned to full activity in an average of 29.1 days, compared with 37.3 days in the K-wire group. No complications were encountered in the implant group, whereas in the K-wire group, complications included broken K-wires, digital deviation, and pin-tract infection. The financial disclosure section of the article reported that the study was funded by the proprietary company that manufactures the implant.

The PhaLinx Hammertoe System (Wright Medical Technology, Inc) includes straight cannulated implants as well as 10-degree angled implants. The cannulation of the straight implant allows the surgeon to cross the MTPJ with a K-wire if additional deformity correction is required across the MTPJ. The implant comes in 4 different sizes, and the set is color-coded to allow for greater ease of use.

The TenFUSE PIPJ implant (Wright Medical Technology, Inc) is a cadaveric, sterilized, partially demineralized allograft with osteoinductive and osteoconductive properties. It is available in straight and 10-degree angled configurations. In a retrospective review by Kominsky and colleagues,[24] 63 PIPJ arthrodesis procedures were performed with the TenFUSE implant. They reported a 97% fusion rate with no complications. Kominsky and colleagues[24] concluded the bone allograft implant was a reliable hammer toe fixation method, which may also aid in the healing process of the fusion site due to osteoinductive properties of the implant. Miller[25] evaluated 26 toes treated with bone allograft pins for fixation of hammertoe contracture. The results of the study showed 1 nonunion, 2 cases of pin fracture, 2 mallet toes, and 3 patients with hyperextension at the MTPJ.

Various investigators have alluded to cost concerns with certain implant technologies. A K-wire typically costs $7 to $15. In comparison, intramedullary implants can cost more than $1000 per implant.[5] With inflating health care costs and the current economic environment, physicians must carefully weigh cost against the benefits of these implant devices. Other disadvantages include difficulty in properly positioning or sizing the implant to adequately correct the digital contracture. If the implant needs to be removed, explantation can be difficult and may neurovascularly compromise the digit. With the use of a K-wire, a malpositioned wire can simply be redirected after placing the digit in the corrected alignment. Meanwhile, implants must be completely removed in cases of malalignment and reinsertion can be difficult. Deep infections are uncommon in hammer toe surgery, and these typically resolve in cases fixated with a K-wire after removal of the K-wire. With the usage of intramedullary implants, however, deep infection requires removal of the implant and sometimes requires the insertion of an antibiotic cement spacer (**Figs. 4** and **5**).

SCREW FIXATION

Cannulated and solid screws are alternative fixation methods for PIPJ arthrodesis. Screws have been inserted in a variety of configurations. The screw can be inserted from the DIPJ and retrograded into the PIPJ. Alternatively, the screw can be inserted from the tip of the distal phalanx and retrograded across both the DIPJ and PIPJ. Cannulated screws allow for placement of a K-wire across the MTPJ. Screws provide compression across the arthrodesis site, potentially yielding higher fusion rates.[20] However, intramedullary screws are subjected to excessive forces that may cause hardware loosening or failure.[20] In the authors' experience, proper placement and purchase of the screw head against the tip of the distal phalanx is technically difficult, but not impossible. This technique is helpful when arthrodesis of the PIPJ and DIPJ is performed simultaneously.

Cannulated intramedullary screws allow for placement of a guide wire across the MTPJ. The guide wire may provide additional stability to the digit throughout the healing process. In the authors' experience, these guide wires are best removed after 4 weeks. These wires are weaker and more flexible than standard 0.045 or 0.062 K-wires, and as a result, they often bend with partial weight bearing. This has caused some surgeons alarm postoperatively; however, we have not had any difficulty removing the bent guide wire, nor have we encountered any residual complications after wire removal. The cannulated screw or cannulated implant in each case has remained stable and intact, providing adequate postoperative permanent fixation.

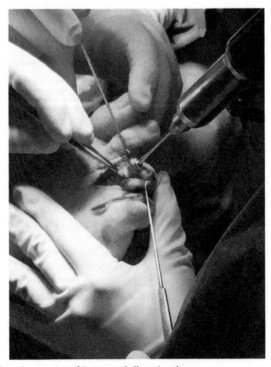

Fig. 4. Reaming for placement of intramedullary implant.

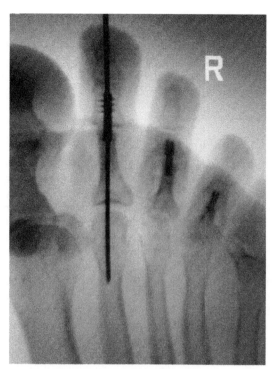

Fig. 5. Single-component cannulated implant in second digit, allowing for K-wire placement through the implant and into the metatarsal head.

Caterini and colleagues[9] described a method using a 3.0-mm titanium screw for PIPJ arthrodesis in which the screw was placed from the distal tip of the toe and retrograded across the DIPJ and PIPJ. The follow-up was 1 to 4 years. During that time, 48 of 51 digits fused, with 3 asymptomatic nonunions. With regard to hardware complications, 7 screws were removed due to persistent pain at the distal tuft of the toe, and 1 screw broke. With this method, however, the placement of the screw violates the DIPJ, rendering the joint immobile. Lane[26] reported on a fixation method in which a 2.0-mm or 3.0-mm cannulated screw was placed through the DIPJ into the middle phalanx and then across the PIPJ. Complications with screw fixation include broken screws, malposition, nail bed protrusion, pain at the distal tuft of the toe, and difficulty of hardware removal.[27]

POSTOPERATIVE CARE

Regardless of the fixation method, the digit is splinted in the corrected position, and the patient may immediately weight bear in a stiff surgical shoe or walking boot. Serial radiographs are performed to evaluate for fusion across the arthrodesis site. If used, the K-wire is removed at 3 to 6 weeks when signs of radiographic fusion are present.

COMPLICATIONS

Complications specific to each method of fixation are discussed in the preceding sections. General complications with regard to PIPJ arthrodesis include recurrence and flail toe. The surgeon should avoid overresecting bone from the interphalangeal joint to avoid a flail toe, but adequate bone should be removed to sufficiently reduce the digital contracture. Flail toe can be a challenging complication. Mahan and colleagues[28] described a technique using bone graft to stabilize a flail toe after hammer toe surgery. Other complications include residual contracture at the MTPJ, contracture at the DIPJ after PIPJ fusion, pseudoarthrosis, nonunion/malunion, infection, prolonged digital swelling, neurologic or vascular compromise to the digit, and hardware failure.[10,11]

SUMMARY

Digital deformities are frequently addressed surgically by foot and ankle surgeons. Fixation options for PIPJ arthrodesis are on the rise. Single K-wire fixation remains the most frequently used form of fixation. K-wires are inexpensive, easy to use, and can be easily removed in cases of malalignment or infection. They can also be placed across the MTPJ for additional sagittal and transverse plane correction.

Absorbable pins offer more permanent stabilization of the PIPJ fusion than K-wires and are slowly resorbed by hydrolysis within the body. They can be trimmed at the tip so that none of the pin protrudes from the skin. They do not, however, provide rotational stability to the digit or compression. They are also more expensive than K-wires.

Screws are also available for PIPJ arthrodesis. They can be placed from the tip of the toe or from the DIPJ into the middle phalanx and are available in cannulated and solid forms. Screws provide compression across the arthrodesis site. Screws placed from the distal tip of the toe may cause hardware irritation at the distal tuft of the digit. Additional concerns include malalignment, cost, and difficulty of hardware removal.

Intramedullary implants include metal and allograft bone implants. These devices require special instrumentation, and insertion techniques vary. Metal implants are

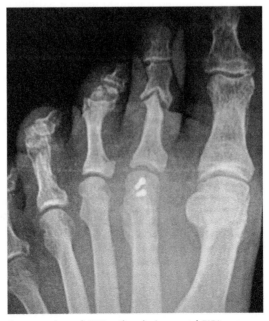

Fig. 6. Asymptomatic nonunion of "V" arthrodesis second PIPJ.

available in single or 2-component designs. Some designs are cannulated to allow a K-wire to be inserted across the MTPJ. These devices have a learning curve and can be prone to malalignment. Cost of intramedullary implants is a tremendous concern, as physician reimbursement is many times less than the cost of the hardware used.

K-wires are very inexpensive compared with intramedullary implants, absorbable pins, and screws, especially if multiple digits are fixated during a single surgical case. The literature shows promise in increased fusion rates and patient satisfaction outcomes with newer technologies, but these novel fixation methods also contribute to increased surgical complexity and overall costs.

Although the literature demonstrates better fusion rates with some alternative fixation methods other than K-wires, this begs the question: is fusion necessary for satisfactory hammer toe repair? Is the goal of PIPJ arthrodesis a fused toe, or is the goal simply a straight, well-aligned, and nonpainful toe? In the authors' experience, many patients are more satisfied with a semirigid asymptomatic nonunion than they are with a rigid digital fusion. Although the radiographs demonstrate a nonunion, the patients are often satisfied. Clearly, a rigid arthrodesis is much less likely to result in a recurrence of the deformity. Usage of the previously mentioned alternative fixation methods yields a more rigid construct, often augmenting the arthrodesis permanently. Nevertheless, it is very difficult to remove screws, absorbable pins, and implants without causing significant destruction to the digit itself. The verdict is still out on which fixation method is best for routine hammer toe repair (**Fig. 6**).

REFERENCES

1. Barnicot N, Hardy R. The position of the hallux in West Africans. J Anat 1995;89: 355–61.
2. DuVries HL. Surgery of the foot. St. Louis: Mosby; 1959. p. 359–60.
3. Lemm M, Green R, Green D. Summary of retrospective long-term review of proximal interphalangeal joint arthroplasty and arthrodesis procedures for hammer toe correction. Reconstructive. Reconstructive Surgery of the Foot and Leg 1996 Update. Tucker (GA): Podiatry Institute Publishing; 1996. p. 193–6.
4. Taylor RG. An operative procedure for the treatment of hammertoe and claw-toe. J Bone Joint Surg 1940;22:608–9.
5. Boffeli TJ, Thompson JC, Tabatt JA. Two-pin fixation of proximal interphalangeal joint fusion for hammertoe correction. J Foot Ankle Surg 2016;55:480–7.
6. Dayton P, Smith D. Dorsal suspension stitch: an alternative stabilization after flexor tenotomy for hammer digit syndrome. J Foot Ankle Surg 2014;53:405–10.
7. Harris W, Mote GA, Malay DS. Fixation of the proximal interphalangeal arthrodesis with the use of an intraosseous loop of stainless-steel wire suture. J Foot Ankle Surg 2009;48:411–4.
8. Konkel KF, Menger AG, Retzlaff SA. Hammer toe correction using an absorbable intramedullary pin. Foot Ankle Int 2007;28:916–20.
9. Caterini R, Farsetti P, Tarantino U, et al. Arthrodesis of the toe joint with an intramedullary cannulated screw for the correction of hammertoe deformity. Foot Ankle Int 2004;25:256–61.
10. Witt BL, Hyer CF. Treatment of hammertoe deformity using a one-piece intramedullary device: a case series. J Foot Ankle Surg 2012;51:450–6.
11. Jay RM, Malay DS, Landsman AS, et al. Dual-component intramedullary implant versus Kirschner wire for proximal interphalangeal joint fusion: a randomized control clinical trial. J Foot Ankle Surg 2016;55(4):697–708.

12. Wilhemi BT, Blackwell SJ, Miller JH, et al. Do not use epinephrine in digital blocks: myth or truth. Plast Reconstr Surg 2001;107(2):393–7.

13. Krunic AL, Wang LC, Soltani K, et al. Digital anesthesia with epinephrine: an old myth revisited. J Am Acad Dermatol 2004;51(5):755–9.

14. D'Angelantonio AM, Nelson-Rinaldi KA, Barnard J, et al. Master techniques in digital arthrodesis. Clin Podiatr Med Surg 2012;29:21–40.

15. Miller JM, Blacklidge DK, Ferdowsian V, et al. Chevron arthrodesis of the interphalangeal joint for hammertoe correction. J Foot Ankle Surg 2010;49:194–6.

16. Reece AT, Stone MH, Young AB. Toe fusion using Kirschner wire fixation: a study of the postoperative infection rate and related problems. J R Coll Surg Edinb 1987;32:158–9.

17. Kramer WC, Parman M, Marks RM. Hammertoe correction with K-wire fixation. Foot Ankle Int 2015;36(5):494–502.

18. Zingas C, Katcherian DA, Wu K. Kirschner wire breakage after surgery of the lesser toes. Foot Ankle Int 1995;16:504–9.

19. Konkel KF, Sover ER, Menger AG, et al. Hammer toe correction using an absorbable pin. Foot Ankle Int 2011;32(1):973–8.

20. Vanore JV. The case against the use of new technologies for hammertoe repair. Reconstructive surgery of the foot and leg. Tucker (GA): Podiatry Institute Publishing; 2013. p. 61–74.

21. Coughlin MJ, Dorris J, Polk E. Operative repair of the fixed hammer toe deformity. Foot Ankle Int 2000;21:94–104.

22. Ellington JK, Anderson RB, Davis WH, et al. Radiographic analysis of proximal interphalangeal joint arthrodesis with an intramedullary fusion device for lesser toe deformities. Foot Ankle Int 2010;31:372–6.

23. Angirasa AK, Barrett MJ, Silvester D. SmartToe™ implant compared with Kirschner wire fixation for hammer digit corrective surgery: a review of 28 patients. J Foot Ankle Surg 2012;51:711–3.

24. Kominsky SJ, Bermudez R, Bannerjee A. Using a bone allograft to fixate proximal interphalangeal joint arthrodesis. Foot Ankle Spec 2013;6(2):132–6.

25. Miller S. Hammer toe correction by arthrodesis of the proximal interphalangeal joint using a cortical bone allograft pin. J Am Podiatr Med Assoc 2002;92:563–9.

26. Lane GD. Lesser digital fusion with a cannulated screw. J Foot Ankle Surg 2005;44:172–3.

27. Fernandez CS, Wagner E, Ortiz C. Lesser toes proximal interphalangeal joint fusion in rigid claw toes. Foot Ankle Clin N Am 2012;17:473–80.

28. Mahan KT, Downey MS, Weinfeld GD. Autogenous bone graft interpositional arthrodesis for correction of flail toe. A retrospective analysis of 22 procedures. J Am Podiatr Med Assoc 2003;93:167–73.

First Metatarsal-Phalangeal Joint Arthrodesis

Primary, Revision, and Salvage of Complications

Thomas S. Roukis, DPM, PhD

KEYWORDS

- Hallux valgus • Hallux rigidus • Fusion techniques • Osteoarthritis • Surgery

KEY POINTS

- First metatarsal-phalangeal joint arthrodesis is a required skill set for foot and ankle surgeons due to its ability to be applied to primary degenerative or rheumatologic arthritis and revision of prior failed surgery to this joint.
- Complications following first metatarsal-phalangeal joint arthrodesis are common following primary intervention and are both more frequent and more severe when revision arthrodesis is performed.
- The development of a nonunion and malunion following first metatarsal-phalangeal joint arthrodesis are predominantly the result of poor surgical technique and can be controlled with surgeon experience and meticulous technique. The use of hand-instrumentation or a crescentic saw to prepare the joint surfaces is preferred over power reamers.
- The use of staples and plates with a compression screw through the plate crossing the arthrodesis site should be avoided to reduce incidence of nonunion. Also, the use of staples and sagittal plane anatomically contoured plates should be avoided to reduce incidence of malunion.
- Plates that combine a thin but mechanically sound contrast, out-of-plane screw orientation, locking and nonlocking screw fixation, and 1 or more eccentric drill slots to afford compression are ideally suited for both primary and revision first metatarsal-phalangeal joint arthrodesis.

INTRODUCTION

Arthrodesis of the first metatarsal-phalangeal joint (MTPJ) has been proposed for treatment of significant first MTPJ pathologic conditions due to the perceived safety and efficacy.[1–3] The author previously undertook a systematic review of electronic databases and other relevant sources to determine the incidence of complications

Department of Orthopaedics, Podiatry and Sports Medicine, Orthopaedic Center, Gundersen Health System, Mail Stop: CO2-006, 1900 South Avenue, La Crosse, WI 54601-5467, USA
E-mail address: tsroukis@gundersenhealth.org

Clin Podiatr Med Surg 34 (2017) 301–314
http://dx.doi.org/10.1016/j.cpm.2017.02.002
0891-8422/17/© 2017 Elsevier Inc. All rights reserved.

following arthrodesis of the first MTPJ.[4] Studies were eligible for inclusion only if they involved patients undergoing arthrodesis of the first MTPJ using modern osteosynthesis techniques (1980 onward time restriction), included a minimum of 30 feet in the publication, evaluated subjects at mean follow-up 12-months or longer duration, included details of complications requiring surgical intervention, and did not involve the use of structural bone graft. Thirty-seven studies involving a total of 2818 first MTPJ arthrodesis procedures were identified that met the inclusion criteria. The weighted mean age of subjects was 59.3 years, follow-up was 34.3 months, and union time was 64.3 days. For those studies that specifically mentioned the indications for first MTPJ arthrodesis, 2656 joints were included as follows (1) severe hallux valgus (47.2%), (2) hallux rigidus (32%), (3) rheumatoid arthritis (11.5%), and (4) revision of failed surgery (9.3%). Joint preparation involved 1 of 3 approaches: (1) hand instrumentation, (2) cup and cone power reamers, and (3) power straight or crescentic saw blades. The arthrodesis osteosynthesis constructs used consisted of 3 broad categories: (1) compression screw fixation, (2) dorsal plate plus or minus oblique compression screw fixation, and (3) staple fixation. Radiographically confirmed nonunion occurred in 5.4% (153 per 2818) with symptomatic nonunion occurring in 32.7% (50 per 153) of these. Salvage of nonunion is complex and involves revision arthrodesis with bulk allograft or autograft, hardware removal, and conversion to a soft-tissue interposition arthroplasty or stemmed prosthetic device, or amputation. Malunion and hardware removal occurred in 6.1% (39 per 640) with dorsal malunion accounting for 87.1% (34 per 39), and the remainder a valgus malunion. Malunion is revised with realignment osteotomy. The incidence of hardware removal was 8.5% (69 per 817). The results of this study have subsequently been independently verified in another systematic review of joint pathologic conditions, preparation technique, and fixation methods for primary first MTPJ arthrodesis.[5] Despite the high union rate with modern osteosynthesis techniques, efforts to reduce the incidence of malunion, hardware removal, and need for salvage following first MTPJ arthrodesis remain warranted.

PRIMARY FIRST METATARSAL-PHALANGEAL ARTHRODESIS

Through a dorsal-medial or direct medial incision the first MTPJ is exposed, followed by resection of the first metatarsal head articular cartilage at the anterior and inferior aspect and the base of the proximal phalanx, with care taken to protect the soft-tissue attachments at the plantar and lateral surfaces to preserve vascularity to the periarticular bone. Due to the higher osseous union rate demonstrated, I prefer to use hand instrumentation to resect the articular cartilage and subchondral bone[5]; however, a crescentic saw blade is useful to create symmetric cup-and-cone surfaces[6] and is simple to perform with minimal cost (**Fig. 1**). I prefer not to use power reamers because these tend to polish sclerotic bone if the subchondral bone plate is not exposed properly, leading to nonunion (**Fig. 2**), especially when combined with locked plate technology (>12% in 2 large series),[7,8] or are too aggressive and resect excessive bone. Concentrated bone marrow aspirate or cancellous bone graft are routinely harvested from the lateral calcaneus to aid in enhancing osseous union because they are simple to obtain and safe to perform.[9,10] For either technique, the surgeon places the index finger on the insertion of the Achilles tendon at the posterior-superior aspect of the calcaneal tuber and the thumb on the origin of the plantar fascia at the inferior aspect of the calcaneal tuber as if using their hand to signal okay. This creates three-fourths of a circle between their index finger, thenar eminence, and thumb, with the remaining one-fourth of the circle being an imaginary line connecting the distal aspects of the

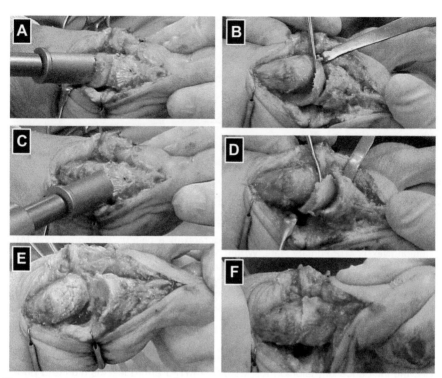

Fig. 1. Intraoperative photographs demonstrating alignment of the crescentic saw blade on the first metatarsal head (*A*) to complete resection of the joint surface, including the metatarsal-sesamoid articulation (*B*). Alignment of the crescentic saw blade on the base of the proximal phalanx (*C*) to complete resection of the joint surface (*D*). The remaining cancellous bone surface has been shingled to increase the surface area for arthrodesis (*E*). Excellent osseous apposition is achieved with this technique (*F*).

index finger and thumb. At a point midway between the distal aspects index finger and thumb along the imaginary line, a 15-gauge needle attached to a 35 mL syringe is advanced through the lateral wall of the calcaneus and into the trabecular bone, followed by slow, steady aspiration of the bone marrow. The needle is redirected every 2 mL to limit dilution of the aspirate. If autogenous graft is required, a 1 cm incision is placed through the skin only. A hemostat is used to dissect to the lateral wall of the calcaneus to clear the adipose and any neurovascular vessels that may be encountered. An 8-mm round-core biopsy trephine is then inserted at a 90° angle to the lateral wall of the calcaneus. The trephine is passed through the lateral wall and into the posterior aspect of the body of the calcaneus until it abuts the medial cortex. This is verified by palpating the medial wall of the calcaneus with the surgeon's nondominant hand. With gentle, gradually increasing circular motions, the trephine is retrieved from the wound. If additional cancellous bone graft is necessary, the trephine is passed through the same hole at different angles rather than new adjacent holes to lessen the risk of an iatrogenic stress riser developing.[11]

The calcaneal bone marrow aspirate or graft is placed within the arthrodesis site and the proximal phalanx of the hallux is compressed against the first metatarsal head to impact the aspirate or graft within the arthrodesis site. The first MTPJ is maintained in a physiologic position dictated by the patient's anatomy but generally consists of slight

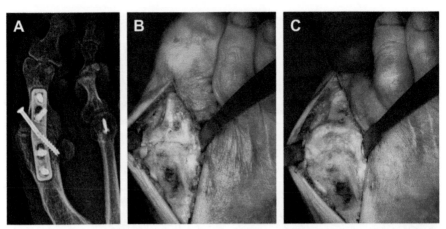

Fig. 2. Anterior-posterior weightbearing radiograph of a painful, misaligned first MTPJ nonunion (NexFix MTP Primary Plate, Wright Medical Technology, Inc, Memphis, TN, USA or Tornier, Bloomington, MN, USA) (*A*). Intraoperative photograph following removal of the internal fixation demonstration the ball-and-socket joint preparation that appears well apposed (*B*). However, great toe plantarflexion reveals an obvious nonunion with sclerotic joint surfaces following use of cup-and-cone power reamers (*C*).

abduction and extension of the hallux with no frontal plane rotation.[2] As noted previously, the incidence of malunion following first MTPJ arthrodesis is high and poorly tolerated. Excessive extension of the hallux will result in a hallux malleus contracture, whereas excessive flexion will result in extension at the hallux interphalangeal joint. Excessive valgus alignment of the hallux will result in abutment with the second toe and the potential for interdigital clavi or development of the crossover second toe deformity. Excessive varus alignment will result in shoe gear –related irritation and the potential for incurvation deformity of the tibial border of the hallux toenail. Therefore, proper intraoperative alignment of the first MTPJ during arthrodesis is essential to minimize malunion complications. The author has found that placing a once-folded 4 inch by 4 inch gauze sponge between the hallux and second toes allows for accurate transverse plane alignment. Similarly, after the foot has been placed up against a sterile instrument tray cover, placing a twice-folded 4 inch by 4 inch gauze sponge underneath the hallux at the level of the hallux interphalangeal joint allows for accurate sagittal plane alignment. There should be no frontal plane rotation, which is easily checked by comparing the dorsal aspect of the hallux toenail with the remaining toes to assure that they are all parallel. With the hallux held in reduced fashion as previously described, a smooth longitudinal Kirchner wire is driven from the tip of the hallux into the first metatarsal to provide provisional fixation but allow for linear compression across the first MTPJ (**Fig. 3**).[12]

Once proper first MTPJ alignment has been confirmed, a compression screw is placed from the base of the proximal phalanx into the first metatarsal head. I prefer to use a larger diameter threaded head cannulated screw to achieve sound compression without prominence. Because the base of the proximal phalanx and first metatarsal head medially have a small surface area and are directly subcutaneous, a headed screw many times lacks sound stability and is prominent, requiring later removal. Additionally, a cadaveric biomechanical study determined that threaded head screws were significantly more stable that headed screws for this indication.[13]

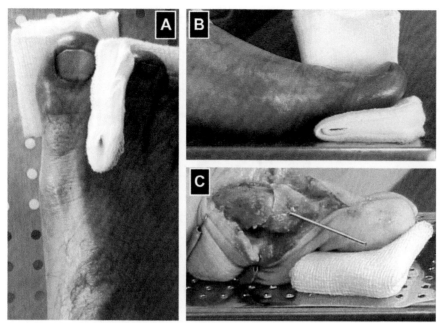

Fig. 3. Dorsal (*A*) and medial view (*B*) of the foot after a 4 inch by 4 inch gauze sponge, which has been folded in half, is placed between the hallux and second toe to properly align the first MTPJ in the transverse plane. Medial view of the foot after a 4 inch by 4 inch gauze sponge, which has been folded in half and then in half again, is placed under the hallux to properly align the first MTPJ in the sagittal plane. Note the foot has been placed against a sterile metallic tray cover during this portion of the procedure, followed by percutaneous placement of a smooth wire obliquely across the first MTPJ (*C*).

Next, a well-contoured dorsal plate is applied because, when combined with an inter-fragmentary screw, it results in a biomechanically stiffer fixation configuration than other technqiues.[14,15] I prefer to use an anatomic, procedure-specific plate that is thin and has a built-in internal eccentric or offset compression drill slot, as well as the ability to use nonlocking and locking screws out of plane to increase construct rigidity (**Fig. 4**). One important consideration is that plates with a hole or slot for a compression screw to cross the arthrodesis site have been demonstrated to have a greater than 30% nonunion and are not recommended for use.[16] The use of a precontoured plate should be used carefully to minimize malunion,[17–19] especially in dorsiflexion, because this markedly increases first metatarsal head planar pressures when excessive dorsiflexion is present.[20,21] I prefer to use single-use, self-contained sterile instrumentation kits and implant packaging (CleanSTART, Novastep, Orangeburg, NY, USA) because no instrument caddies or sterilization is required, allowing them to be used on demand, and because this reduces the sterile field overload. There is no risk of having damaged or missing instruments, operating room costs are reduced, the implants are easily tracked, and the operating room turn-over time is reduced.

The surgical site is then irrigated, closed in layers, and a well-padded dressing applied about the forefoot. Patients perform immediate weightbearing in a stiff-soled postoperative shoe, emphasizing weight on the heel and lateral forefoot. Postoperative radiographs are obtained at 8 weeks to verify osseous union. If any concern

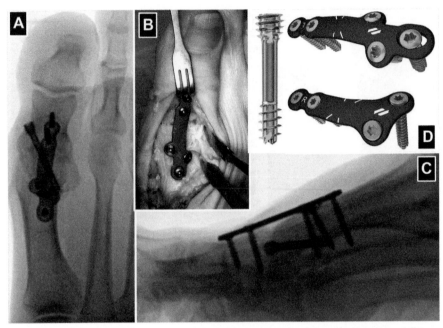

Fig. 4. Anterior-posterior fluoroscopic (*A*) and intraoperative (*B*), as well as lateral fluoroscopic (*C*) images following primary first MTPJ arthrodesis with a threaded head compression screw and specially designed plate. Schematic representations of the specific threaded head Nexis 4 mm screw (*left*) and standard (*top*) and short (*bottom*) Airlock MTP arthrodesis plates (Novastep, Orangeburg, NY, USA) used (*D*). Note that this patient also underwent revision second toe proximal interphalangeal joint arthrodesis (Lync 10° Offset Hammertoe System, Novastep, Orangeburg, NY, USA) and Weil shortening third metatarsal osteotomy (Nexis 2.3 mm Snap-off Screw, Novastep, Orangeburg, NY, USA). (*Courtesy of* Novastep, Orangeburg, NY; with permission.)

for delayed union exists, serial radiographs are obtained until radiographic and clinic signs of arthrodesis exist.

REVISION FIRST METATARSAL-PHALANGEAL ARTHRODESIS

A basic principle of any revision surgery is to use the original incision and to minimize undermining. I prefer to use a sharp curved handled osteotome to elevate the soft-tissues off of the underlying hardware or implant and bone because it's more robust, easier to hold, and comes in a variety of widths, allowing the surgeon to elevate a larger volume of soft-tissue than a traditional periosteal elevator. Straight and curved rongeurs, osteotomes and mallet, curettes, and power rotary burrs are used to resect any ectopic bone engulfing the prior internal fixation or prosthetic components. Once identified, the internal fixation is removed, with care taken to limit stripping the screw heads because this complicates the remainder of the surgery. The old adages, "no one looks good removing hardware" and "it takes either 5 minutes or 55 minutes to remove hardware" are unfortunately true. As such, it is important to anticipate problems removing internal fixation hardware, especially if screws are cold-welded to the plate fixation, and to have the correct screwdrivers, screw extraction instrument sets, a hollow-mill set to core over the screws, a variety of pliers, as well as carbide drills and high-speed metal cutting tools to facilitate extraction.[22,23] Prosthetic components can usually be freed from the underlying bone, preserving maximum bone; however, on occasion, the metallic components require osteotomy and complete excision with a mantle of bone that leaves a massive osseous defect (**Fig. 5**). Whenever possible, I prefer to use hand instrumentation to prepare the remaining bone surfaces to minimize thermal injury and control the bone resection better than when power instruments are used.[24] Although allogenic corticocancellous[25] and trabecular metal blocks[26] are available for use to bridge the osseous gaps present, I prefer autogenous bone graft whenever the osseous defect is greater than 1.5 cm because autograft reliably results in an osseous union. A systematic review previously conducted by the author regarding the incidence of nonunion after autogenous iliac crest bone block distraction salvage arthrodesis of the first MTPJ revealed the incidence of nonunion was only 4.8%.[27] Subsequent publications verify the high union rate with autogenous iliac crest bone block distraction salvage arthrodesis of the first MTPJ.[28–33] It can be difficult to achieve proper position of the first MTPJ arthrodesis when a large bone block is used because the toe seems to toggle around like a marionette along with the bone graft. To minimize this, I have found it helpful to temporarily pin the bone graft to the second metatarsal with multiple Steinman pins while deciding on the best contouring configuration for the proximal and distal segments of the bone graft and native bone. I prefer to contour the ends of the bone graft using hand instrumentation; however, the cup-and-cone reamers applied slowly and with the bone graft soundly secured on the back table can be useful in precisely shaping the ends of the bone graft.[34,35] Once the bone graft and native bone has been properly contoured, the graft is packed tightly with the bone marrow aspirate concentrate and/or cryopreserved bone cellular matrix to augment osseous union.[36] Osteosynthesis primarily consists of a well-contoured dorsal plate (**Fig. 6**), ideally specifically intended for revision first MTPJ arthrodesis situations, including flanges that wrap the proximal phalanx and first metatarsal shafts to increase fixation options; built-in internal compression slots, including the ability to secure the interposed bone graft; and the ability to use large diameter, out-of-plane nonlocking and locking screws.[33,37–39] If the remaining bone is insufficient and precludes plate fixation, external fixation[40] or multiple axially placed Steinman pin fixation[41] remain viable options.

The surgical site is then irrigated, closed in layers, and a well-padded dressing applied about the forefoot with patients maintained nonweightbearing for 8 to 16 weeks until postoperative radiographs and/or computerized-tomography scan verifies osseous union. In these situations, because osseous union is frequently delayed, serial radiographs are obtained until radiographic and clinical signs of arthrodesis exist.

SALVAGE OF FAILED FIRST METATARSAL-PHALANGEAL ARTHRODESIS

A malunited first MTPJ arthrodesis is best addressed by removal of the internal fixation and either a crescentic saw osteotomy[42] at the apex of the deformity to allow for triplane correction or an opening wedge osteotomy[43] if additional length is required.

Hallux interphalangeal arthritis associated with a first MTPJ arthrodesis can be treated with arthrodesis of the hallux interphalangeal joint, resection of the first MTPJ arthrodesis, and conversion to an interpositional arthroplasty[44] or arthrodesis of the hallux interphalangeal joint alone.[45]

There are situations in which revision of a failed first MTPJ arthrodesis with bone block distraction arthrodesis is simply not feasible due to hostile soft-tissues, concern for vascular embarrassment with any appreciable lengthening, or inability to remain

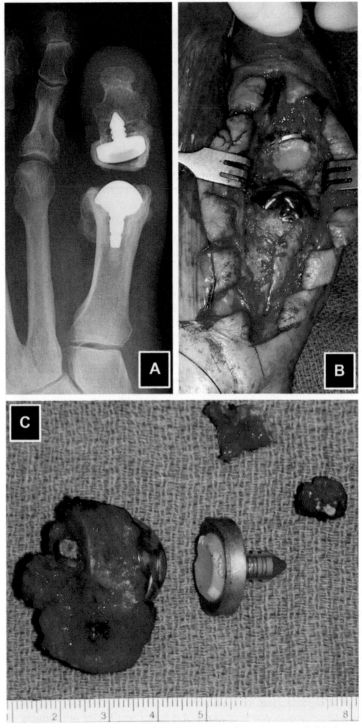

Fig. 5. Anterior-posterior radiograph (*A*) and intraoperative photograph (*B*) demonstrating severe subsidence of a 2-component cemented first MTPJ prosthesis (Kinetic Great Toe

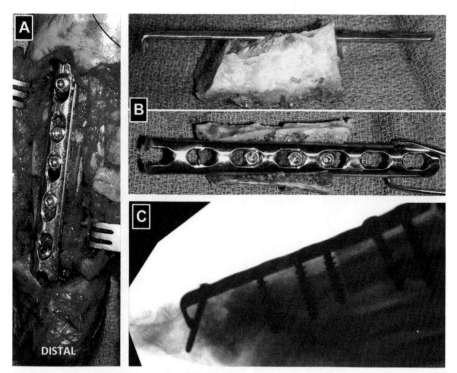

Fig. 6. Intraoperative photograph (A) following implantation of the tricortical autogenous anterior iliac crest bone graft secured to a one-third tubular straight plate (B; side and top views) that has been contoured distally into a hook-shape due to the limited bone stock available for purchase in the distal phalanx, as demonstrated on lateral fluoroscopic imaging (C).

nonweightbearing for an extended period. In these situations, if the resected bone is minimal, removal of the retained internal fixation and conversion to a soft-tissue interpositional arthroplasty by leaving the fibrous tissue encompassing the metallic implants intact and purse-stringing it,[46] or placing a collagen sponge within the resected joint,[47] have been demonstrated to be successful. Alternatively, removal of the internal fixation and implantation of a stemmed prosthesis plus or minus metallic grommets can relieve pain and maintain function (**Fig. 7**).[48,49] In situations in which massive nonreconstructable osseous defects or deep infection are present, partial first ray amputation (**Fig. 8**) with an in-shoe orthosis with toe filler should be considered.[48]

Implant, Kinetikos Medical Inc, Carlsbad, CA, USA). Note that multiple Z-plasty incisions have been placed along the first ray incision to accommodate for the anticipated first ray length gained with the distraction arthrodesis performed. Intraoperative photograph of the explanted prosthetic components demonstrating the significant volume of bone, requiring resection from the first metatarsal segment due to the extensive amount of polymethylmethacrylate cement used (C).

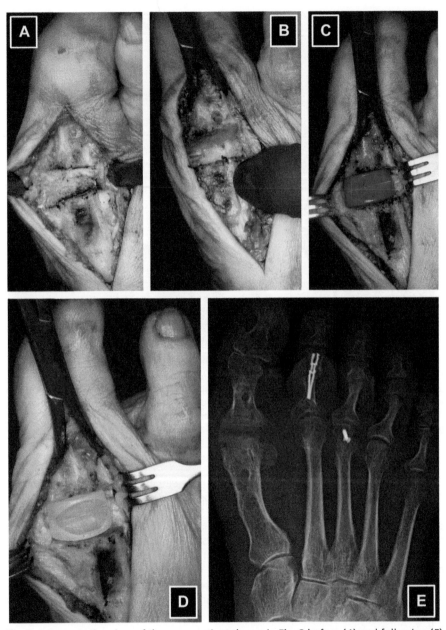

Fig. 7. Intraoperative view of the same patient shown in **Fig. 2** before (*A*) and following (*B*) corrective freehand joint resection to accommodate a total prosthetic stemmed implant arthroplasty (*C*; trial component). Intraoperative (*D*) and anterior-posterior weightbearing radiograph (*E*) following total prosthetic stemmed implant arthroplasty (Classic Flexible Great Toe Implant, Integra, Plainsboro, NJ, USA).

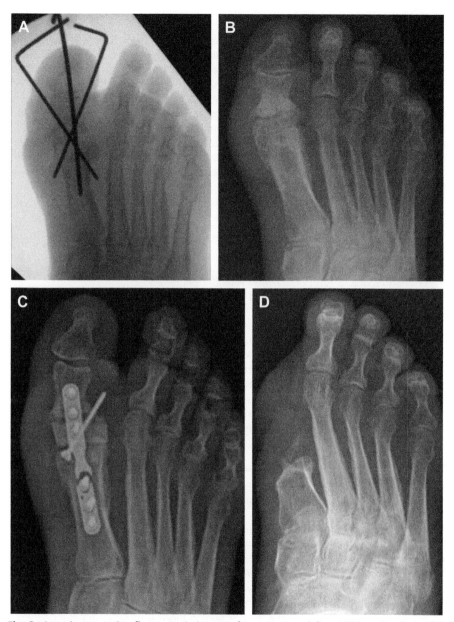

Fig. 8. Anterior-posterior fluoroscopic image of an attempted first MTPJ arthrodesis with multiple crossed Steinman pin fixation (*A*) that predictably led to a nonunion and persistent pain (*B*). Anterior-posterior weightbearing radiograph following a failed attempt at revision first MTPJ arthrodesis with an allograft bone block and dorsal mini-fragment plate and oblique compression screw (MTPJ Plate, Trimed, Inc, Santa Clarita, CA, USA) that developed a deep space abscess and osteomyelitis (*C*). Note the fractured plate, migrated headed oblique screw and obvious nonunion between the host bone and interposed allograft. The patient underwent a successful partial first ray amputation as a salvage procedure (*D*).

SUMMARY

Primary and revision first MTPJ arthrodesis are valuable procedures for myriad first MTPJ pathologic conditions, leading to significant improvement in pain and function. However, nonunion, malunion, and painful internal fixation are common complications frequently requiring secondary surgical intervention. Poor surgeon joint preparation technique and positioning, as well as use of internal fixation systems with design flaws should be avoided to minimize complications associated with primary and revision first MTPJ arthrodesis. Salvage techniques are few, are both costly and complicated to perform, and carry a higher incidence of complications than primary arthrodesis efforts. Therefore, first MTPJ arthrodesis mandates proper attention to detail regarding joint preparation technique, positioning, osteosynthesis, and postoperative care to minimize complications and patient suffering.

REFERENCES

1. Coughlin MJ. Arthrodesis of the first metatarsophalangeal joint. Orthop Rev 1990; 29:177–86.
2. Yu GV, Shook JE. Arthrodesis of the first metatarsophalangeal joint: current recommendations. J Am Podiatr Med Assoc 1994;84:266–80.
3. Marks RM. Arthrodesis of the first metatarsophalangeal joint. Instr Course Lect 2005;54:263–8.
4. Roukis TS. Nonunion after arthrodesis of the first metatarsal-phalangeal joint: a systematic review. J Foot Ankle Surg 2011;50:710–3.
5. Korim MT, Mahadevan D, Ghosh A, et al. Effect of joint pathology, surface preparation and fixation methods on union frequency after first metatarsophalangeal joint arthrodesis: a systematic review of the English literature. Foot Ankle Surg 2016. http://dx.doi.org/10.1016/j.fas.2016.05.317.
6. Shute GC, Sferra JJ. Use of the crescentic saw for arthrodesis of the first metatarsophalangeal joint. Foot Ankle Int 1998;19:719–20.
7. Ellington JK, Jones CP, Cohen BE, et al. Review of 107 hallux MTP joint arthrodesis using dome-shaped reamers and a stainless-steel dorsal plate. Foot Ankle Int 2010;31(5):385–90.
8. Hunt KJ, Ellington JK, Anderson RB, et al. Locked versus nonlocked plate fixation for hallux MTP arthrodesis. Foot Ankle Int 2011;32:704–9.
9. Schade VL, Roukis TS. Percutaneous bone marrow aspirate and bone graft harvesting techniques in the lower extremity. Clin Podiatr Med Surg 2008;25:733–42.
10. Roukis TS, Hyer CF, Philbin TM, et al. Complications associated with autogenous bone marrow aspirate harvest from the lower extremity: an observational cohort study. J Foot Ankle Surg 2009;48:668–71.
11. Roukis TS. A simple technique for harvesting autogenous bone grafts from the calcaneus. Foot Ankle Int 2006;27:998–9.
12. Roukis TS. A simple technique for positioning the first metatarsophalangeal joint during arthrodesis. J Foot Ankle Surg 2006;45:56–7.
13. Rongstad KM, Miller GJ, Vander Griend RA, et al. A biomechanical comparison of four fixation methods of first metatarsophalangeal joint arthrodesis. Foot Ankle Int 1994;15:415–9.
14. Politi J, Hayes J, Njus G, et al. First metatarsal-phalangeal joint arthrodesis: a biomechanical assessment of stability. Foot Ankle Int 2003;24:332–7.
15. Buranosky DJ, Taylor DT, Sage RA, et al. First metatarsophalangeal joint arthrodesis: quantitative mechanical testing of six-hole dorsal plate versus crossed screw fixation in cadaveric specimens. J Foot Ankle Surg 2001;40:208–13.

16. Gross C, Bei C, Gay T, et al. A short-term retrospective of first metatarsophalangeal joint arthrodesis using a plate with pocketlock fixation. Foot Ankle Spec 2015;8:466–71.
17. DeOrio JK. Technique tip: arthrodesis of the first metatarsophalangeal joint–prevention of excessive dorsiflexion. Foot Ankle Int 2007;28:746–7.
18. Leaseburg JT, DeOrio JK, Shapiro SA. Radiographic correlation of hallux MP fusion position and plate angle. Foot Ankle Int 2009;30:873–6.
19. Marsland D, Konan S, Eleftheriou K, et al. Fusion of the first metatarsophalangeal joint: precontoured or straight plate? J Foot Ankle Surg 2016;55:509–12.
20. Bayomy AF, Aubin PM, Sangeorzan BJ, et al. Arthrodesis of the first metatarsophalangeal joint: a robotic cadaver study of the dorsiflexion angle. J Bone Joint Surg Am 2010;92:1754–64.
21. Alentorn-Geli E, Gil S, Bascuas I, et al. Correlation of dorsiflexion angle and plantar pressure following arthrodesis of the first metatarsophalangeal joint. Foot Ankle Int 2013;34:504–11.
22. Hak DJ, McElvany M. Removal of broken hardware. J Am Acad Orthop Surg 2008;16:113–20.
23. Kumar G, Dunlop C. Case report: a technique to remove a jammed locking screw from a locking plate. Clin Orthop Rel Res 2011;469:613–6.
24. Singh B, Draeger R, Del Gaizo DJ, et al. Changes in length of the first ray with two different first MTP fusion techniques: a cadaveric study. Foot Ankle Int 2008;29: 722–5.
25. Luk PC, Johnson JE, McCormick JJ, et al. First metatarsophalangeal joint arthrodesis technique with interposition allograft bone block. Foot Ankle Int 2015;36: 936–43.
26. Sagherian BH, Claridge RJ. Porous tantalum as a structural graft in foot and ankle surgery. Foot Ankle Int 2012;33:179–89.
27. Mankovecky MR, Prissel MA, Roukis TS. Incidence of nonunion of first metatarsal–phalangeal joint arthrodesis with autogenous iliac crest bone graft after failed Keller-Brandes arthroplasty: a systematic review. J Foot Ankle Surg 2013; 52:53–5.
28. Garras DN, Durinka JB, Bercik M, et al. Conversion arthrodesis for failed first metatarsophalangeal joint hemiarthroplasty. Foot Ankle Int 2013;34:1227–32.
29. Gross CE, Hsu AR, Lin J, et al. Revision MTP arthrodesis for failed MTP arthroplasty. Foot Ankle Spec 2013;6:471–8.
30. Malhotra K, Nunn T, Qamar F, et al. Interposition bone block arthrodesis for revision hallux metatarsophalangeal joint surgery: a case series. Foot Ankle Int 2015; 36:556–64.
31. Lareau CR, Deren ME, Fantry A, et al. Does autogenous bone graft work? A logistic regression analysis of data from 159 papers in the foot and ankle literature. Foot Ankle Surg 2015;21:150–9.
32. Feranec M, Hart R. Distraction arthrodesis of the 1st metatarsophalangeal joint. Foot Ankle Surg 2016;22:92.
33. Loewy EM, Clare MP. First MTP joint distraction arthrodesis with cancellous autograft and bridge plating: a novel surgical technique to restore maximum length. Tech Foot Ankle Surg 2016;15:103–9.
34. Whalen JL. Clinical tip: interpositional bone graft for first MP fusion. Foot Ankle Int 2009;30:160–2.
35. Ahluwalia RS, Blucher NC, Platt SR, et al. Creative cutting to contour and correct Hallux bone graft for three planes of correction. Foot Ankle Surg 2013;19: 199–201.

36. Anderson J, Jeppesen N, Hansen M, et al. First metatarsophalangeal joint arthrodesis: comparison of mesenchymal stem cell allograft versus autogenous bone graft fusion rates. Surg Sci 2013;4:263–7.

37. Bhosale A, Munoruth A, Blundell C, et al. Complex primary arthrodesis of the first metatarsophalangeal joint after bone loss. Foot Ankle Int 2011;32:968–72.

38. Schuh R, Trnka HJ. First metatarsophalangeal arthrodesis for severe bone loss. Foot Ankle Clin 2011;16:13–20.

39. Aiyer AA, Myerson MS, Dall G, et al. The biomechanical evaluation of revision first metatarsophalangeal arthrodesis: a cadaveric study. Foot Ankle Spec 2015;8: 369–77.

40. Schweinberger MH, Roukis TS. Salvage of the first ray with external fixation in the high-risk patient. Foot Ankle Spec 2008;1:210–3.

41. Smith RW, Joanis TL, Maxwell PD. Great toe metatarsophalangeal joint arthrodesis: a user-friendly technique. Foot Ankle Int 1992;13:367–77.

42. Geppert MJ. Sagittal plane correction of a malunited first metatarsophalangeal arthrodesis utilizing a crescentic osteotomy. Foot Ankle Int 1997;18:102.

43. Cullen NP, Angel J, Singh D, et al. Clinical tip: revision first metatarsophalangeal joint arthrodesis for sagittal plane malunion with an opening wedge osteotomy using a small fragment block plate. Foot Ankle Int 2005;26(11):1001–4.

44. Babazadeh S, Su D, Blackney MC. Hallux IP arthritis after MP arthrodesis managed with interpositional arthroplasty of MP joint and IP fusion: case report. Foot Ankle Int 2011;32(9):900–4.

45. Mizel MS, Alvarez RG, Fink BR, et al. Ipsilateral arthrodesis of the metatarsophalangeal and interphalangeal joints of the hallux. Foot Ankle Int 2006;27:804–7.

46. Hope M, Savva N, Whitehouse S, et al. Is it necessary to re-fuse a non-union of a hallux metatarsophalangeal joint arthrodesis? Foot Ankle Int 2010;31:662–9.

47. Heller E, Robinson D. Gelfoam first metatarsophalangeal replacement/interposition arthroplasty: a case series with functional outcomes. Foot 2011;21:119–23.

48. Sung W, Weil LS, Weil LS Sr, et al. Total first metatarsophalangeal joint implant arthroplasty: a 30-year retrospective. Clin Podiatr Med Surg 2011;28:755–61.

49. Kumar V, Clough T. Silastic arthroplasty of the first metatarsophalangeal joint as salvage for failed revisional fusion with interpositional structural bone graft. BMJ case Rep 2013. http://dx.doi.org/10.1136/bcr-2013-008993.

Tarsometatarsal Arthrodesis for Lisfranc Injuries

Nicholas J. Bevilacqua, DPM

KEYWORDS

- Lisfranc injuries • Fracture dislocation • Ligamentous injury
- Primary arthrodesis tarsometatarsal joint

KEY POINTS

- Open reduction and internal fixation has traditionally been the treatment of choice for most Lisfranc fracture-dislocations.
- A trend toward primary fusion is seen, especially for purely ligamentous injuries.
- Consideration should be made for primary fusion in select fracture-dislocations cases.
- In select Lisfranc injuries, quality anatomic reduction and primary arthrodesis will result in a stable foot and, over time, it will remain stable with predictable results and less need for secondary surgery.

INTRODUCTION

The Lisfranc joint, also known as the tarsometatarsal joint, is part of the structural support of the transverse arch of the midfoot. Injuries to this joint complex represent approximately 0.2% of all fractures. Traumatic injuries to the tarsometatarsal joint complex can be devastating and often associated with long-term disability from subsequent painful post-traumatic osteoarthritis and deformity.[1,2]

Treatment concepts have evolved over the years. Surgical treatment traditionally consisted of closed reduction and immobilization or closed reduction and percutaneous fixation.[3] These methods were unsuccessful in most cases.[1,4] Closed reduction often did not result in anatomic alignment due to interposed soft tissue and/or fracture fragments, and casting did not provide the adequate restraint to resist further displacement. This often resulted in repeat dislocation, residual midfoot instability, and limited functionality. As a result, the proposed management of Lisfranc injuries progressed toward open reduction and internal fixation (ORIF) and this remains the current preferred management.[1]

Foot and Ankle Surgery, North Jersey Orthopaedic Specialists, 730 Palisade Avenue, Teaneck, NJ 07666, USA
E-mail address: Nicholas.bevilacqua@gmail.com

Clin Podiatr Med Surg 34 (2017) 315–325
http://dx.doi.org/10.1016/j.cpm.2017.02.003
0891-8422/17/© 2017 Elsevier Inc. All rights reserved.
podiatric.theclinics.com

Although ORIF is the mainstay of treatment, patient results often deteriorate over time. Post-traumatic degenerative changes resulting in pain and deformity are common with Lisfranc injuries.[1,5] Even with anatomic reduction and stable internal fixation, results are often suboptimal. Arthrodesis of the affected joints is a well-accepted salvage procedure and, consequently, primary arthrodesis has been proposed for both Lisfranc fracture-dislocations and ligamentous Lisfranc injuries.[1,6,7] This article reviews the indications, technique, and outcomes of primary arthrodesis for Lisfranc injuries.

ANATOMY

The Lisfranc joint is part of the structural support of the transverse arch of the midfoot. Knowledge of the anatomy is essential for understanding injury patterns. This joint includes the 3 cuneiforms, the cuboid, and the bases of the 5 metatarsals. From a functional standpoint, this joint complex is often divided into 3 columns. The medial column (first metatarsal cuneiform joint), the middle column (second and third metatarsal cuneiform joint and the articulations between the middle and lateral cuneiform), and the lateral column (fourth and fifth metatarsal cuboid joint).[2,8]

The anatomic shape of the transverse arch of the midfoot provides inherent structural stability and additional support is offered by strong ligamentous attachments. Dorsal, plantar, and interosseous ligaments join the metatarsals together to form an extensive ligamentous support network with the exception being between the first and second metatarsals. Instead, there is the Lisfranc ligament, an interosseous ligament that runs obliquely from the medial cuneiform to the base of the second metatarsal. Studies have shown this ligament to be the strongest in the tarsometatarsal complex.[8] The plantar ligaments are stronger than the dorsal ligaments.

Although the columns function interdependently, the motion of each is different.[8] The lateral column allows for the most movement in the sagittal plane with an average of 13 mm, whereas there is almost no movement in the middle column (only 0.8 mm of movement in this plane). There is approximately 3.5 mm of sagittal plane motion in the medial column.[8,9] These differences in sagittal plane motion between the 3 columns have implications in the injury pattern and treatment.

The relatively immobile medial and central columns have been referred to as nonessential joints,[1] whereas the more mobile lateral column is considered essential. Obtaining stability of the medial column and maintaining motion in lateral column is vital for optimal outcomes when treating injuries to the tarsometatarsal complex.

MECHANISM OF INJURY

It is important to note the different mechanisms of injury to the tarsometatarsal joint complex.[8] A host of mechanisms have been described, ranging from high-energy crush injuries to low-energy twisting injuries. Low-energy injuries may result in subtle injuries that are difficult to diagnose and are distinctly different than high-energy injuries, which are usually obvious and may result in comminuted, intra-articular fractures (**Fig. 1**).

Numerous classifications have been proposed based on mechanism of injury, direction of force, and resultant injury pattern. Quenu and Kuss[10] first proposed a classification for Lisfranc injuries and organized them into 3 groups: homolateral, isolated, and divergent. This was later modified by Hardcastle and colleagues,[3] and further refined by Myerson and colleagues.[11] The Myerson-modified Hardcastle classification system is a more detailed system and has been shown to be reliable and may be used

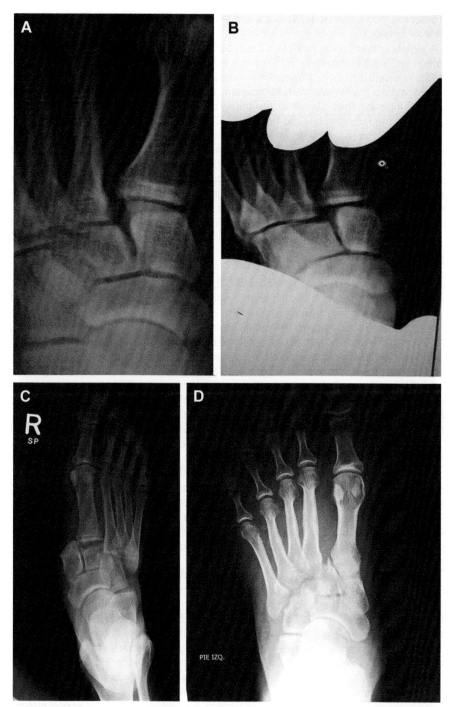

Fig. 1. (*A*) Subtle ligamentous injury seen on anteroposterior weightbearing radiographs. (*B*) Confirmed instability with stress radiographs. (*C*) Obvious ligamentous injury. (*D*) Obvious fracture-dislocation injury.

in outcome studies and to provide standard terminology among clinicians for tarsome-tatarsal injuries.[12]

A simple classification has been described and divides these injuries into 2 basic categories: subtle and obvious.[13] The subtle injuries have no obvious fracture or diastasis, whereas the obvious fractures involve a visible fracture of any portion of the Lisfranc complex. Nunley and Vertullo[14] created a classification system to address subtle Lisfranc injuries. They classified the injury based on clinical examination findings, weightbearing radiographs, and bone scans.

A pragmatic approach is to divide Lisfranc injuries into the purely ligamentous injuries and fracture-dislocations. Purely ligamentous injuries of the tarsometatarsal joint complex pose a therapeutic challenge. Suboptimal outcomes are consistently reported even after anatomic reduction and stabilization.[15] Between 40% and 94% of these patients develop post-traumatic degeneration requiring secondary arthrodesis.[6,7,15–17] Ly and Coetzee[7] reported better short-term and medium-term outcomes with primary arthrodesis compared with ORIF of ligamentous Lisfranc joint injuries.[7]

INDICATIONS FOR ARTHRODESIS

ORIF has been the mainstay of treatment of Lisfranc injuries; however, as noted, inferior results have been reported in patients with primarily ligamentous injuries. Kuo and colleagues[17] evaluated the outcome of ORIF of Lisfranc injuries in 48 subjects with an average follow-up of 4 years. The purely ligamentous subgroup had worse outcomes despite initial anatomic reductions and internal fixation.

Recently, the trend has been moving toward primary fusion for purely ligamentous injuries. In a prospective, randomized clinical trial, Ly and Coetzee[7] compared primary arthrodesis with traditional ORIF for the treatment of primary ligamentous Lisfranc injuries. Forty-one subjects with an isolated ligamentous Lisfranc injury were enrolled and 20 subjects were treated with ORIF and 21 subjects were treated with primary arthrodesis of the medial 2 or 3 rays. Seventy-five percent of subjects who underwent ORIF had displayed some degree of loss of correction and degenerative joint changes at the final follow-up of 42.5 months postoperatively. Five subjects in the ORIF group had persistent pain and were eventually treated with arthrodesis. At 2 years, their results revealed a mean American Orthopaedic Foot and Ankle Society midfoot score of 68.6 points in the ORIF group compared with 88 points in the primary fusion group. They found that the group treated with primary fusion had more rapid recovery, and a superior return to function. As a result, they concluded that primary stable arthrodesis provides better short-term and medium-term outcomes than ORIF in primary ligamentous injuries.

In a comparable prospective, randomized study, Henning and colleagues[1] compared the outcomes of subjects treated with primary arthrodesis to those treated with ORIF for acute Lisfranc injuries. Their study found no significant difference in functional outcomes, clinical assessment, and subject satisfaction between the 2 groups. A secondary aim of the study was to determine whether there was a difference in secondary surgeries. The rate of secondary surgeries between the ORIF and primary arthrodesis groups were 78.6% and 16.7%, respectively. This difference was significant and not surprising because routine screw removal was built into the study.

Secondary surgery, specifically hardware removal, is very common after ORIF of Lisfranc injuries.[18] When transarticular fixation is used, removing the screw creates large osteochondral defects on both sides of the joint. The high incidence of post-traumatic degeneration post-ORIF and screw removal may be attributed to this type of fixation. More recently, a trend has been seen for ORIF using dorsal bridging locking plates.[18] Dorsal bridge plating stabilizes the joints and, unlike transarticular screws, do not need to be passed through the articular cartilage. Also, dorsal bridge plating may be used to span comminuted fractures and stabilize the joint when screw fixation is not possible (**Fig. 2**).

Although dorsal bridge plating requires more dissection during placement and implant removal, it leads to similar results compared with transarticular fixation in terms of functional outcomes and patient satisfaction.[19] Bridge plates have been designed to be temporary and if the hardware remains after ORIF it is essentially a nonunion. Lau and colleagues[18] compared outcomes for 3 different methods of fixation: screw fixation, dorsal plating, and combination of plate and screws, and found a similar rate of hardware removal for all (86%, 82%, and 82%, respectively). Therefore, the surgeon should consider the increased rate of hardware removal along with its associated morbidities following ORIF.[20]

After ORIF of severe intra-articular fractures and subsequent hardware removal, incomplete or complete autofusion may occur across the joints and, in cases of partial or incomplete fusion, salvage arthrodesis may be necessary. In cases of severe, intra-articular fractures (especially when using dorsal bridge plating for ORIF), the surgeon may consider primary fusion with dorsal plates. This will potentially obviate hardware removal and salvage fusion. Some surgeons argue against primary fusion because of the required dissection; however, with the trend moving toward dorsal bridge plating, the amount of dissection is very similar.

In fracture-dislocations of the tarsometatarsal joint complex where there are 2 large fragments at the base of the second metatarsal, with the Lisfranc ligament being

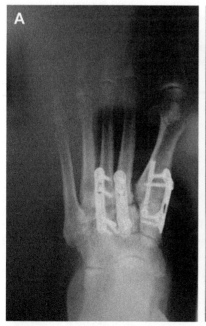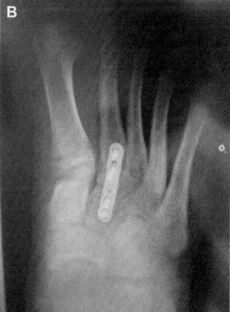

Fig. 2. (*A*) Dorsal bridge plating fixation for ORIF Lisfranc fracture dislocation. (*B*) Dorsal bridge plate used for ORIF of second tarsometatarsal joint. Two large fragments at the base of the second metatarsal, with the Lisfranc ligament being attached to 1 of the fragments. The plate allowed for maintains of reduction and avoided transarticular fixation.

attached to 1 of the fragments, fixation may provide stability.[21] However, in cases with more comminution, it is unlikely that ORIF will reconstruct the joint without subsequent degeneration. In these cases, primary arthrodesis should be considered. Fusion outcomes will remain stable, whereas ORIF results will likely deteriorate over time as post-traumatic arthritis develops.

The relatively immobile medial and central columns have been referred to as nonessential joints[1] and, therefore, arthrodesis will not affect the long-term function. Losing the comparatively small amount of motion available at the tarsometatarsal joints will be less critical to altering the foot biomechanics. The author considers primary arthrodesis in select cases of acute injuries to the tarsometatarsal joint complex; particularly in purely ligamentous and severe intra-articular communicated fractures.

Arthrodesis of the tarsometatarsal joint is also considered in the neglected Lisfranc injury. In this situation, procedures may include arthrodesis in situ or arthrodesis with a realignment midfoot osteotomy (**Fig. 3**).

SURGICAL TECHNIQUE

After appropriate workup and medical optimization patients are scheduled for operative management. Primary arthrodesis for Lisfranc injuries should be delayed until the soft tissue envelope normalizes and is conducive to surgical intervention. Radiographs, including anteroposterior, lateral, and medial oblique views of the foot, are obtained and computed tomography studies may be obtained to aid in surgical planning and used to evaluate the extent of injury. The medial and central nonessential joints are anatomically reduced and fused while the more mobile essential lateral column is reduced and temporarily fixated.

Patients are then brought into the operating room and placed supine on the operating room table. A bump may be placed under the ipsilateral hip to correct external rotation to improve access to the dorsal foot. A well-padded calf tourniquet is applied; however, a thigh tourniquet may be used, especially if tibial bone graft is considered. The operative extremity is prepared and draped in the usual manner.

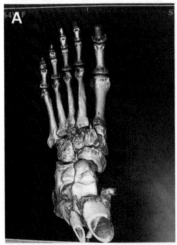 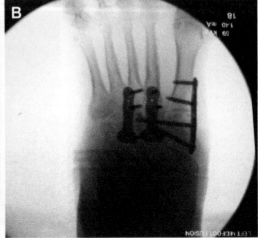

Fig. 3. (*A*) Late treatment of Lisfranc fracture dislocation. Computed tomography used to further evaluate the extent of injury. (*B*) Primary fusion of medial and central columns for definitive management of neglected Lisfranc injury.

A 2-incisional dorsal approach is used. The medial incision is used to expose the first tarsometatarsal joint and is placed on the dorsal aspect of the joint. The lateral incision is used to access the second and third tarsometatarsal joints and is placed between the joints or slightly more lateral to maximize the skin bridge. Variation in incision placement is common and depends on injury pattern. The incisions may be shifted more medial or lateral depending on joint involvement. Intraoperative fluoroscopy may be used to verify appropriate incision placement and to confirm access to affected joints.

The medial incision is carefully dissected down through the subcutaneous tissue layers. The extensor hallucis longus tendon is identified and retracted safely. The joint is identified by manipulating the first metatarsal and a capsular incision is made. The joint is prepared for primary arthrodesis using a combination of curettes, osteotomes, and rongeur. The tarsometatarsal joints are deep, ranging from 2.5 to 3.0 cm, and it is imperative to remove all of the cartilage. The subchondral plate is fenestrated using a 2.0-mm drill. The medial aspect of the second tarsometatarsal joint may be accessed through this incision but, if not, the lateral incision is made. It is imperative to limit aggressive skin retraction and excessive handling of the superficial skin edges. Meticulous dissection is performed and the dorsalis pedis artery and the deep peroneal nerve are identified and retracted safely. The second metatarsal is manipulated and the joint is identified. This keystone joint is recessed and will be more proximal relative to the first. Interposed soft tissue is excised and small fracture fragments may be removed to aide in reduction. The joint and the articulation between the first and second metatarsal bases are prepared in a similar fashion as the first tarsometatarsal joint. Attention is then directed to the third tarsometatarsal joint and the joint is identified and prepared for fusion in a similar manner. All cartilage is removed and the subchondral plate is fenestrated.

The first tarsometatarsal is reduced and fixated. A significant factor in achieving superior radiologic and functional outcomes after surgery is the quality of the anatomic reduction.[18] The windlass mechanism may be used to assist in anatomic reduction. The first metatarsal is aligned to the medial cuneiform and provisionally fixated with Kirschner (K)-wires or guide wires from the cannulated screw set. A variety of different fixation techniques have been described for stabilization of the tarsometatarsal fusion, including plates and screws, lag screws, and staples.[22] Biomechanical models have shown dorsal plates to provide stable constructs and maintain anatomic reduction.[18,23] If the first metatarsal is amendable to screw fixation, typically 2 crossed screws are used. The screws are inserted with a lag technique for compression. A compression screw and locking plate combination may be used as well.

Anatomic reduction of the second and third tarsometatarsal joint are performed. The second metatarsal is aligned to the middle cuneiform and lateral base of the first and the third metatarsal is aligned to the lateral cuneiform. The joints are provisionally fixated with K-wires and the forefoot is palpated to ensure the metatarsal heads are balanced. The first metatarsal (sesamoids) should be slightly plantar relative to the second. Fluoroscopy is used to verify alignment. Definitive fixation is achieved with either a single screw directed from distal to proximal or a dorsal locking plate. In purely ligamentous injuries, screw fixation often achieves adequate compression and stability. In these cases, a cannulated 4.0-mm lag screw or a 3.5-mm cortical screw placed in lag technique allows for adequate compression and stability. However, in cases in which there is significant commuted intra-articular fracture fragments and not amenable to screw fixation, a dorsal locking plate is used (**Fig. 4**).

The stability is assessed intraoperatively under fluoroscopy and, if there is a gap between the first and second metatarsal bases, it is reduced using bone reduction

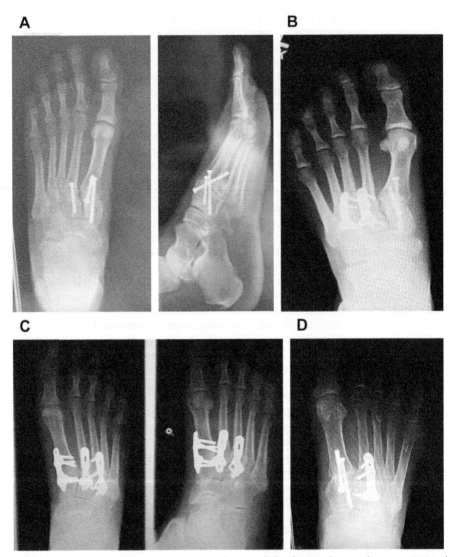

Fig. 4. (*A*) Screw fixation used for primary fusion of the first and second tarsometatarsal joint. (*B*) Screw fixation for primary arthrodesis of first tarsometatarsal joint and dorsal plate fixation used for fusion of comminuted, intra-articular fractures of the second and third tarsometatarsal joints. (*C*) Plate fixation used for primary arthrodesis of medial and central columns. (*D*) Screw fixation used for primary fusion of first tarsometatarsal and dorsal bridge plate used for primary fusion of comminuted fracture of second tarsometatarsal.

forceps and fixated. This screw is not placed if the region is markedly stable in the sagittal plane because a fused medial column will typically prevent subsequent displacement in the transverse plane.[2]

If the injury involves the lateral column and the joint is deemed unstable, it is anatomically reduced and fixated to the cuboid with K-wires. Fusion of the lateral column should be avoided. Mulier and colleagues[24] compared ORIF of severe Lisfranc injuries with partial and complete fusion. At 30-month follow-up, subjects who underwent complete fusion (including lateral column) had more pain than the ORIF and partial arthrodesis groups (which had a similar level of pain).[21,24] Fluoroscopy is used to confirm reduction, alignment, and fixation.

Careful layered closure is performed. The capsule overlying the tarsometatarsal joints and the subcutaneous tissue are closed with absorbable suture and the skin is closed with nylon with minimal tension. The wound is dressed and patients are placed in a bulky compressive dressing; a posterior splint is applied in the operating room and patients are nonweightbearing with crutches or may use a knee scooter. The splint is removed at 2 weeks and, if indicated, sutures are removed. Patients are then placed in a well-padded short leg fiberglass cast and remain nonweightbearing. At 4 weeks, radiographs are taken and if progression toward healing is noted, patients are placed in a removable boot and toe-touch weightbearing is permitted. Otherwise, if no progression is noted, the patient remains nonweightbearing. Progressive weightbearing is typically permitted between 6 and 12 weeks in a removable boot and, if radiographs confirm healing, patients are weaned out of the boot and ambulate in normal footwear at 12 weeks. The K-wires in the lateral column are usually removed 6 to 8 weeks postoperatively.

OUTCOMES AFTER TARSOMETATARSAL FUSION

Precise anatomic reduction and primary arthrodesis for certain Lisfranc injuries will result in a stable foot and, over time, will remain stable with predictable results. Patients tolerate fusion of the relatively immobile medial and central columns. Losing the comparatively small amount of motion available at the tarsometatarsal joints will be less critical to altering the foot biomechanics. Mulier and colleagues[24] reviewed 28 subjects with severe, acute Lisfranc injuries treated with ORIF, partial fusion or complete fusion. The study showed that subjects tolerated partial fusion and no difference was found between the ORIF group and the partial arthrodesis group. Subjects who underwent complete fusion yielded the poorest results. The nonunion rate was low in fusion group. It was suggested that the high fusion rate after primary fusion may be due to the hyperemia that follows the severe injury, although surgeon experience also plays a role.[15] Given that the nonunion rate was low in the arthrodesis group, this may be a factor in deciding to proceed with primary arthrodesis rather than ORIF in select cases.

Sheibani-Rad and colleagues[15] performed a systematic review of 6 studies with 193 subjects comparing primary arthrodesis and ORIF. They found a mean American Orthopaedic Foot and Ankle Society score of 72.5 and 88.0 for ORIF and arthrodesis patients, respectively. Complications following fusion included pseudarthrosis, painful hardware, nonunion, and delayed union. They concluded that both procedures can yield satisfactory and equivalent results, although primary arthrodesis might hold a slight advantage for these injuries in terms of clinical outcomes.

In a retrospective review of young subjects following primary partial arthrodesis for Lisfranc injuries, MacMahon and colleagues[25] found that most subjects were able to return to their previous physical activities, many of which were high-impact. However, some subjects experienced some postoperative limitations in exercise. Myerson and Cerrato[8] do not recommend primary arthrodesis for athletes because they believe maintenance of motion in the medial column, as well as limited motion in the middle column, is necessary to restore full function in these patients.

Although post-traumatic osteoarthritis of the tarsometatarsal joints is not an issue following primary fusion, adjacent joint arthritis may be. Loss of motion may lead to an overload of the adjacent joints in the midfoot.[26] Reinhardt and colleagues[27] reported a 12% rate of adjacent joint arthritis 42 months on average after primary fusion.

SUMMARY

Much controversy exists for the ideal treatment of Lisfranc injuries. ORIF has traditionally been the treatment of choice for most Lisfranc fracture-dislocations. A trend toward primary fusion is seen, especially for purely ligamentous injuries. Consideration should be made for primary fusion in select fracture-dislocations cases. In select Lisfranc injuries, quality anatomic reduction and primary arthrodesis will result in a stable foot and, over time, will remain stable with predictable results with less need for secondary surgery.

REFERENCES

1. Henning JA, Jones CB, Sietsema DL, et al. Open reduction internal fixation versus primary arthrodesis for lisfranc injuries: a prospective randomized study. Foot Ankle Int 2009;30(10):913–22.
2. Boffeli TJ, Pfannenstein RR, Thompson JC. Combined medial column primary arthrodesis, middle column open reduction internal fixation, and lateral column pinning for treatment of Lisfranc fracture-dislocation injuries. J Foot Ankle Surg 2014;53(5):657–63.
3. Hardcastle PH, Reschauer R, Kutscha-Lissberg E, et al. Injuries to the tarsometatarsal joint. Incidence, classification and treatment. J Bone Joint Surg Br 1982; 64(3):349–56.
4. Arntz CT, Hansen ST Jr. Dislocations and fracture dislocations of the tarsometatarsal joints. Orthop Clin North Am 1987;18(1):105–14.
5. Arntz CT, Veith RG, Hansen ST Jr. Fractures and fracture-dislocations of the tarsometatarsal joint. J Bone Joint Surg Am 1988;70(2):173–81.
6. Sangeorzan BJ, Veith RG, Hansen ST Jr, et al. Salvage of Lisfranc's tarsometatarsal joint by arthrodesis. Foot Ankle 1990;10(4):193–200.
7. Ly TV, Coetzee JC. Treatment of primarily ligamentous Lisfranc joint injuries: primary arthrodesis compared with open reduction and internal fixation. A prospective, randomized study. J Bone Joint Surg Am 2006;88(3):514–20.
8. Myerson MS, Cerrato RA. Current management of tarsometatarsal injuries in the athlete. J Bone Joint Surg Am 2008;90(11):2522–33.
9. Ouzounian TJ, Shereff MJ. In vitro determination of midfoot motion. Foot Ankle 1989;10(3):140–6.
10. Quenu E, Kuss G. Etude sur les luxations du metatarse. Rev Chir 1909;39(1).
11. Myerson MS, Fisher RT, Burgess AR, et al. Fracture dislocations of the tarsometatarsal joints: end results correlated with pathology and treatment. Foot Ankle 1986;6(5):225–42.
12. Mahmoud S, Hamad F, Riaz M, et al. Reliability of the Lisfranc injury radiological classification (Myerson-modified Hardcastle classification system). Int Orthop 2015;39(11):2215–8.
13. Spitalny A. Lisfranc and midfoot fractures. In: Fractures of the foot and ankle. Philadelphia: Elsevier Saunders; 2004. p. 95–141.
14. Nunley JA, Vertullo CJ. Classification, investigation, and management of midfoot sprains: Lisfranc injuries in the athlete. Am J Sports Med 2002;30(6):871–8.
15. Sheibani-Rad S, Coetzee JC, Giveans MR, et al. Arthrodesis versus ORIF for Lisfranc fractures. Orthopedics 2012;35(6):e868–73.

16. Buzzard BM, Briggs PJ. Surgical management of acute tarsometatarsal fracture dislocation in the adult. Clin Orthop Relat Res 1998;(353):125–33.

17. Kuo RS, Tejwani NC, Digiovanni CW, et al. Outcome after open reduction and internal fixation of Lisfranc joint injuries. J Bone Joint Surg Am 2000;82-A(11): 1609–18.

18. Lau S, Howells N, Millar M, et al. Plates, screws, or combination? radiologic outcomes after lisfranc fracture dislocation. J Foot Ankle Surg 2016;55(4):799–802.

19. Hu SJ, Chang SM, Li XH, et al. Outcome comparison of Lisfranc injuries treated through dorsal plate fixation versus screw fixation. Acta Ortop Bras 2014;22(6): 315–20.

20. Smith N, Stone C, Furey A. Does open reduction and internal fixation versus primary arthrodesis improve patient outcomes for Lisfranc trauma? A systematic review and meta-analysis. Clin Orthop Relat Res 2016;474(6):1445–52.

21. Eleftheriou KI, Rosenfeld PF. Lisfranc injury in the athlete: evidence supporting management from sprain to fracture dislocation. Foot Ankle Clin 2013;18(2): 219–36.

22. Withey CJ, Murphy AL, Horner R. Tarsometatarsal joint arthrodesis with trephine joint resection and dowel calcaneal bone graft. J Foot Ankle Surg 2014;53(2): 243–7.

23. Bayley E, Duncan N, Taylor A. The use of locking plates in complex midfoot fractures. Ann R Coll Surg Engl 2012;94(8):593–6.

24. Mulier T, Reynders P, Dereymaeker G, et al. Severe Lisfrancs injuries: primary arthrodesis or ORIF? Foot Ankle Int 2002;23(10):902–5.

25. MacMahon A, Kim P, Levine DS, et al. Return to sports and physical activities after primary partial arthrodesis for Lisfranc injuries in young patients. Foot Ankle Int 2016;37(4):355–62.

26. Abbasian MR, Paradies F, Weber M, et al. Temporary internal fixation for ligamentous and osseous Lisfranc injuries: outcome and technical tip. Foot Ankle Int 2015;36(8):976–83.

27. Reinhardt KR, Oh LS, Schottel P, et al. Treatment of Lisfranc fracture-dislocations with primary partial arthrodesis. Foot Ankle Int 2012;33(1):50–6.

Subtalar Joint Arthrodesis for Elective and Posttraumatic Foot and Ankle Deformities

 CrossMark

Lawrence A. DiDomenico, DPM[a,b,c,*],
Danielle N. Butto, DPM, AACFAS[d]

KEYWORDS

- Posttraumatic osteoarthritis subtalar joint • Subtalar joint arthrodesis
- Foot and ankle deformities

KEY POINTS

- Identify the appropriate patient who suffers from posttraumatic subtalar joint osteoarthritis.
- Joint preparation is very important and most time should be spent preparing the joint for arthrodesis.
- Fixation construct needs to be done very well and effectively to provide a solid Arbeitsgemeinschaft für Osteosynthesefragen (AO) construct for good results.

Subtalar joint arthrodesis is a procedure used in posttraumatic arthritis, osteoarthritis, tarsal coalition management, posterior tibial tendon dysfunction, and inflammatory arthropathies.[1,2] It also can be used in deformity correction before or at the same time as total ankle arthroplasty and is incorporated in the tibial-talocalcaneal fusion. The goals of the procedure are to eliminate pain, improve function, restore stability, and realign the rearfoot.[1] The procedure has high patient satisfaction with low complications, while preserving motion in adjacent tarsal joints.[1,3] Union rates are reported from 84% to 100%.[1,2,4] Screw removal is reported between 13% and 22%[4] (**Fig. 1**).

This article discusses the use of the subtalar joint arthrodesis in both elective and posttraumatic foot and ankle deformities.

Disclosure Statement: There is no conflict with my consulting and business relationships as it pertains to this article.
[a] Northside Hospital, Youngstown, OH, USA; [b] Ankle and Foot Care Centers, KSU College of Podiatric Medicine, 8175 Market Street, Youngstown, OH 44512, USA; [c] St. Elizabeth Hospital, Youngstown, OH, USA; [d] St. Francis Hospital and Medical Center, Hartford, CT, USA
* Corresponding author. 8175 Market Street, Youngstown, OH 44512.
E-mail address: LD5353@aol.com

Clin Podiatr Med Surg 34 (2017) 327–338
http://dx.doi.org/10.1016/j.cpm.2017.02.004
0891-8422/17/© 2017 Elsevier Inc. All rights reserved.

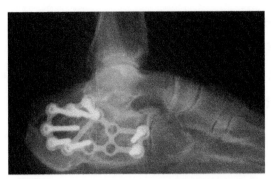

Fig. 1. A lateral radiograph projection demonstrating posttraumatic subtalar joint arthritis secondary to an unsuccessful open reduction internal fixation of a calcaneal fracture. Note the decrease in the calcaneal inclination angle, thus the talus sits more parallel to the ground instead of in a declination along and parallel to the first metatarsal. This change of the talar position also causes changes at the tibial talar joint where abutment of the talus occurs on dorsiflexion of the ankle. This impacts the ankle joint and will cause a limitation in range of motion at the ankle joint secondary to the position of the talus relative to the calcaneus.

ANATOMY AND BIOMECHANICS

The subtalar joint is composed of the dorsal surface of the calcaneus and the plantar surface of the talus. There are 3 facets on each surface: anterior, middle, and posterior. The posterior facet of the calcaneus is the largest of the 3.[5] The sinus tarsi is located laterally as the end point of the sulcus tali and sulcus calcanei. The sulcus tali and calcanei form the sulcus tali in which the interosseus talocalcaneal ligament lies. The bifurcate and cervical ligaments along with the inferior extensor retinaculum insert on the sinus tarsi.[3,6]

The subtalar joint has both an extraosseous and intraosseous blood supply. The extraosseous blood supply to the subtalar joint comes from the posterior tibial artery, the anterior tibial artery, and the peroneal artery. The posterior tibial artery gives branches that anastomose with branches from the anterior tibial artery and the peroneal artery. The posterior tibial artery also gives off a branch known as the artery of the tarsal canal. The artery of the tarsal canal gives off a large branch to the talar body and smaller branches to the calcaneus. Additionally, in anastomoses with the artery of the sinus tarsi. The intraosseous blood supply centers around the talus. The talar head is supplied by the dorsalis pedis and the artery of the sinus tarsi. The main bloody supply to the body of the talus is from the anastomoses between the artery of the tarsal canal and branches of the dorsalis pedis. The body receives additional blood supply from the deltoid branch of the artery of the tarsal canal. The calcaneus and navicular have a rich vascular connection with the talus through intraosseous ligaments and the joint capsule.[5]

The subtalar joint is responsible for the conversion of rotatory forces of the lower extremity and dictates the movement of the midtarsal joint. The subtalar joint moves as a single unit around a single joint axis. The joint axis is oriented 42° form the horizontal plane and 16° from the sagittal plane oriented obliquely posterior-plantar-lateral to anterior-dorsal-medial. The joint exhibits triplanar motion.[5] Movement in the frontal plane occurs along the longitudinal/sagittal axis producing inversion and eversion. A 2:1 ratio of supination to pronation is considered "normal." Movement in the transverse plane occurs along the vertical component of the axis. This movement is referred to as abduction and adduction. Movement in the sagittal plane occurs along the frontal component of the axis, producing dorsiflexion and plantarflexion. The motion in the 3 planes occurs simultaneously, producing pronation or supination. Pronation consists of eversion, abduction, and dorsiflexion. Supination consists of inversion, adduction, and plantarflexion.[5]

PATHOLOGY
Posttraumatic Arthritis

A well-known complication status post calcaneal fracture is subtalar joint arthritis. When the fracture is not primarily fixated, deformities, including an incongruous subtalar joint, decreased calcaneal height, lateral calcaneal wall widening, calcaneal-fibular abutment, peroneal tendon impingement, and hindfoot varus/valgus can ensue. The subtalar joint arthrodesis can be used to realign the rearfoot and decrease these postoperative complications while eliminating pain. In cases of decreased calcaneal height, an osteotomy or bone graft will have to be used to restore the height. One method is subtalar distraction bone block fusion. The talar and calcaneal joint surfaces are prepared for fusion. A lamina spreader is used to distract the subtalar joint to the appropriate height and also the surgeon needs to be sure the frontal plane is in neutral to slight valgus. A tricortical bone graft is then inserted. Two fully threaded large cancellous screws are then placed through the graft and across the joint[7] (**Figs. 2** and **3**).

Osteoarthritis/Inflammatory Arthritis

When arthritis, either osteo or inflammatory, is present in the subtalar joint that is painful and limits hindfoot function, a subtalar joint arthrodesis is warranted when bracing fails. The arthrodesis can be performed isolated if degenerative changes are isolated or in combination with a talonavicular, calcaneal-cuboid, or other midfoot arthrodesis procedures when degenerative changes are more widespread. Astion and colleagues[8] in a cadaveric study simulated arthrodesis of the subtalar joint. They found that 26% of the motion in the talonavicular joint and 56% of the motion of the

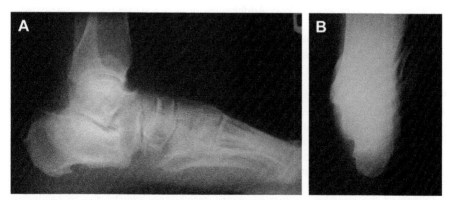

Fig. 2. A lateral and calcaneal axial preoperative radiograph projections in a patient who suffered a calcaneal fracture. (*A*) Lateral radiograph: Note the decrease in the calcaneal inclination angle, the subsequent change in Meary angle, secondary changes at the tibial talar joint, posttraumatic osteoarthritis, and malalignment of the subtalar joint. (*B*) Calcaneal axial: Note the widening of the calcaneus secondary to a lateral wall expansion and mild varus deformity.

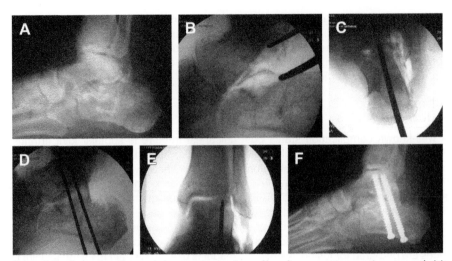

Fig. 3. (A) A lateral radiograph in a patient who suffers from posttraumatic osteoarthritis secondary to a calcaneal fracture. (B) A intraoperative view demonstrating a lamina spreader being used to expose the subtalar joint for preparation of a tricortical cancellous bone graft. The lamina spreader is also used for getting the heel out of varus and into a neutral position. (C) An intraoperative calcaneal axial view following exostectomy of the lateral wall of the calcaneus to prevent lateral impingement symptoms. The guide wires for 2 large fully threaded cancellous screws are inserted in preparation for the fixation. (D) An intraoperative lateral fluoroscopic view is used to assess the position of the tricortical cancellous bone graft and guide wires in preparation for 2 large fully threaded positional screws to be inserted. Please note the angular changes of the talus with the tricortical cancellous bone graft in place. (E) An intraoperative ankle anteroposterior fluoroscopic view that is used to be sure the guide pins and screws do not enter the ankle joint. (F) A postoperative lateral radiographic projection demonstrating changes in the talus position as well as good incorporation of a tricortical cancellous bone graft with 2 large fully threaded positional screws.

calcaneocuboid joint was retained. Additionally, 46% of the excursion of the posterior tibial tendon was retained.

When the talonavicular joint is added to the arthrodesis, the motion of the remaining joints is limited to about 2° and the excursion of the posterior tibial tendon was limited to 25% of the preoperative value.[8]

Coalition

A tarsal coalition is a congenital bridging between 2 or more tarsal bones. It is the most common cause of peroneal spastic flat foot. A subtalar joint coalition can occur between either the anterior, middle, or posterior facets, but the middle facet is the most common.[9] Subtalar joint coalitions commonly present between the ages of 12 and 16 but can also be seen in the adult population.[10] When conservative measures fail, surgical options include resection of the coalition or arthrodesis. Unfortunately, resection of the coalition seldom produces satisfactory results due to secondary degenerative changes that develop over time (**Fig. 4**).

Posterior Tibial Tendon Dysfunction

Posterior tibial tendon dysfunction leads to pes planus deformity. The deformity is hallmarked by lateral column shortening, talar head uncovering, hyperpronation of the

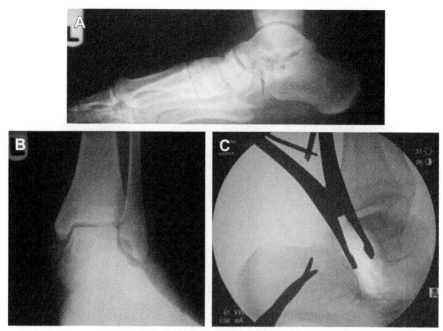

Fig. 4. (A) This is a lateral radiograph of a patient who suffers from a painful flatfoot secondary to a middle facet talocalcaneal coalition. Note the changes of in the calcaneal pitch, the secondary changes of the navicular cuneiform joint, and elevation of the first metatarsal relative to the talus. (B) An ankle radiograph demonstrating a patient who suffers from a painful flatfoot deformity secondary to a middle facet talocalcaneal medial coalition. Note the exposure of the talar head medially and valgus deformity of the hindfoot. (C) An intraoperative lateral projection demonstrating a lamina spreader distracting the subtalar joint from a medial approach for a middle facet talocalcaneal coalition. The lamina spreader allows exposure to the subtalar joint and assists the surgeon in aligning the subtalar joint into a neutral position.

subtalar joint, and valgus position of the calcaneus.[11] Fusion procedures are indicated in the stage III and stage IV pes planus deformity. In contrast to the triple arthrodesis, which has a high rate of progression of ankle joint arthritis, the isolated subtalar joint spares 26% of the talonavicular joint motion, 50% of the calcaneal-cuboid joint motion, and 46% of posterior tibial tendon excursion.[3] With proper positioning, the isolated subtalar joint arthrodesis resolves hindfoot valgus, eliminates hyperpronation, and restores the talo-first metatarsal angle (**Fig. 5**).

Ankle Pathology

When osteoarthritis is present in both the subtalar joint and ankle, the surgeon may elect to perform a tibio-talocalcaneal joint fusion. This is typically fixated with an intramedullary nail or a femoral locking plate.[12] Additionally, the subtalar joint arthrodesis may be added to achieve proper rearfoot alignment before or in conjunction with total ankle arthroplasty. The hindfoot must be in rectus alignment to prevent failure of the implant.

PHYSICAL EXAMINATION

The initial examination of any patient with suspected subtalar joint pathology should include vascular assessment and neurology examination, including assessing for

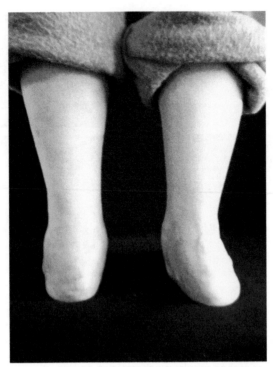

Fig. 5. A clinical view of a patient who suffers from posterior tibial tendon dysfunction. This patient has postoperative reconstruction consisting of the left subtalar joint arthrodesis left and preoperative right. Note the alignment difference once the subtalar joint in positioned appropriately.

positive Tinel sign. The subtalar joint range of motion should be assessed with the patient in the prone position. Normal subtalar joint range of motion includes 2:1 inversion to eversion. Rigid, limited range of motion may be indicative of a coalition. The position of the rearfoot should be assessed for valgus position of the heel. A valgus position may present in posterior tibial tendon dysfunction and in coalition. Peroneal spasm is a strong indication of coalition.

RADIOGRAPHIC EXAMINATION

Anteroposterior, lateral, and oblique radiographs of the foot should be taken. Angles to examine include the calcaneal inclination angle, Meary angle, and Kite angle. With subtalar joint arthritis, one may encounter a decrease in calcaneal inclination while the Kite and Meary angles are increased. If the patient had previously sustained a calcaneal fracture the Gissane and Bohler angles should be examined. An increased Gissane angle and decreased Bohler angle suggest loss of height within the posterior facet. A lateral radiograph can be used to examine for a middle facet talocalcaneal coalition. A middle facet talocalcaneal coalition is suspected when a "halo-sign" is present inferior to the subtalar joint. In addition, specialty views can be taken to further examine the subtalar joint. An oblique lateral view can be taken to view the anterior joint. The medial aspect of the foot is placed on the film and the foot is inclined 45° to the film. The X-ray tube is centered 1 inch below and 1 inch anterior to the lateral malleolus. A medial oblique axial can be taken to view the middle facet. The foot is dorsiflexed then inverted. The leg is medially rotated 60° and the foot is rested on a 30° wedge and the tube is directed axially 1 inch anterior and 1 inch below the lateral malleolus. The lateral oblique axial is used to visualize the posterior facet. The foot is dorsiflexed and everted. The limb is laterally rotated 60° and rested on a 30° wedge. The tube is directed axially and centered 1 inch below the medial malleolus (Isherwood). These specialized views can be tricky to take and some imaging centers may not offer these views. In these cases, advanced imaging, such as computed tomography (CT) and/or MRI may need to be ordered. A CT may be particularly advantageous in cases of posttraumatic arthritis. An MRI can be useful in the cases in which coalition is suspected.

CONSERVATIVE TREATMENT

Conservative measures should be prescribed before surgery is considered. Oral nonsteroidal anti-inflammatories or topical compounding creams can be used for inflammatory control. Depending on the degree of deformity, orthotics may be useful to control hindfoot motion. If the deformity is more severe, bracing with an ankle-foot orthosis may be considered. Diagnostic injections into the sinus tarsi can be used. If the diagnostic block is successful, steroid can be added to the mixture to control intra-articular inflammation. When activities of daily living are affected by chronic subtalar joint pain, surgical intervention is warranted.

SURGICAL MANAGEMENT

The patient is placed in the supine position with a hip bump. Choice of incision placement is based on the pathology. A commonly used incision is the lateral sinus tarsi incision. The incision extends from the distal fibula distally to the calcaneocuboid joint. A lateral extensile incision may be preferred if the patient has had previous calcaneal fracture fixation. Sharp and blunt is then used to penetrate down to the subcutaneous issues. One must take care to visualize and retract the sural nerve if encountered. The deep fascia and extensor retinaculum are then identified. The subtalar joint should then be manipulated to identify the sinus tarsi and the lateral process of the talus. The deep fascia, extensor digitorum muscle belly, and periosteum are then dissected free to expose the sinus tarsi and the posterior facet. The sinus tarsi is then evacuated of its contents. Cartilage is resected from talar and calcaneal articular surfaces. When resecting cartilage along the medial aspect of the posterior facet, care should be taken to avoid the medial neurovascular structures.

If rearfoot position must be corrected, a bone wedge can be removed. The base of the resected wedge would be placed laterally for correction of rearfoot varus, while a medially based wedge would resect to correct rearfoot valgus.[3] Another option would be adding an autograft or allograft wedge to correct the hindfoot position.[11] The joint is then positioned in a neutral position while cupping the heel or dorsiflexing the foot. The guide pin is placed and subtalar joint position is assessed under fluoroscopy. Fixation techniques vary from single screw fixation to double. Additionally, the screws can be placed in a variety of orientations. A biomechanical study by Hungerer and colleagues[13] revealed that a delta configuration of the screws resulted in the greatest biomechanical stiffness with the lowest deflection of the arthrodesis. They found no significant difference between use of a 6.5-mm or 8.0-mm screw. The authors prefer to use large cannulated screws. A drain can be placed if deemed necessary.

Fusion can also be achieved arthroscopically. Lateral decubitus position is ideal for access via the anterolateral and posterolateral portals. A 2.7-mm scope is used to visualize the subtalar joint. A shaver is used to remove all synovitis and burr, shavers, and curettes are used to remove all the cartilage.[14]

In cases of loss of height, incongruity, or severe malalignment in the subtalar joint, bone grafting may be necessary. A curvilinear incision parallel and posterior to the peroneal tendons is used.[15] A longitudinal, posterior incision may be used in a subtalar joint distraction to protect the soft tissues. This is especially useful when the anterior, medial, and/or lateral soft tissues have been violated from prior surgical attempts, local infection, or high-energy fractures.[16] A lamina spreader is placed in to the posterior subtalar joint and positioned to both distract the subtalar joint to the desired height as well as correct any frontal plane deformity if present. In more severe cases, a medial-based external fixator can be applied to help with distraction and allowing the subtalar joint to be placed in a neutral position. The resultant wedge is measured and a cortico-cancellous wedge is then cut and contoured to fit the void. Once placed and fixated, the remaining voids are tightly packed with crushed allograft, autograft, or bone substitutes depending on surgeon preference[15] (**Fig. 6**).

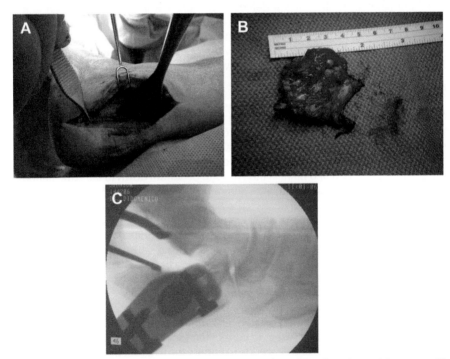

Fig. 6. (*A*) A posterior lateral approach for a patient who suffered a calcaneal fracture with significant height loss. The posterior lateral approach is used to protect the soft tissues when using a large tricortical cancellous bone graft for distraction of the subtalar joint. Because of the naturally occurring skin lines, the distraction causes less injury to the soft tissues posteriorly than it does laterally. (*B*) Image depicting an exostectomy of the lateral wall of the calcaneus to be used as an autogenous bone graft. Any remaining soft tissue attachments are removed and the bone is prepared in a bone mill to be morselized for later bone grafting. (*C*) An intraoperative lateral fluoroscopic view demonstrating a medial-based external fixator and lamina spreader used to address a varus deformity of the subtalar joint. The lamina spreader and external fixator maintain the position of the subtalar joint, as well assist with exposure while preparing the joint and inserting the tricortical cancellous bone graft.

In cases of severe pes planus deformity, a subtalar joint arthrodesis may be combined with a talonavicular arthrodesis. In these cases, the surgeon may choose to use an isolated medial double approach rather than fusing the subtalar joint from the lateral approach. A curvilinear incision starts at the medial malleolus and comes out toward the plantar talonavicular joint. Care is taken to preserve the deltoid ligaments. Advantages to the procedure include direct visualization and easier manipulation to adequately reduce the displaced heel back underneath the talus with clear exposure to joint preparation for fusion.[17]

No matter the approach or technique, hindfoot alignment should be checked intraoperatively with a calcaneal-axial view before final fixation is achieved. In some cases, a posterior calcaneal osteotomy may need to be combined with the subtalar joint fusion to reduce varus or valgus. Once adequate reduction of the deformity is achieved, fixation can be introduced. The types, size, and configuration of screws varies among surgeons. In a biomechanical evaluation of subtalar fusion, Hungerer and colleagues[13] assessed various screw configurations and types. They examined screws placed parallel, counter-parallel, and in a delta configuration. Additionally, they examined cannulated, partially threaded, and solid screws in both 6.5-mm and 8.0-mm screws. Their results found that the delta configuration resulted in the greatest biomechanical stiffness and lowest degree of deflection. Increasing the screw size from 6.5 to 8.0 mm resulted in no additional stability. Additionally, there was no statistical significance between solid and partially threaded cannulated screws (**Figs. 7–9**).

FIXATION

Typically, 2 large cancellous screws are used in the subtalar joint when attempting an arthrodesis. The screws are either partially threaded or fully threaded based on the goal of the surgery. With an attempt to perform a subtalar joint arthrodesis, the authors advocate using 2 partially threaded large cancellous screws. The partially threaded cancellous screws will accomplish internal compression within the subtalar joint. In cases in which the goal is to perform a subtalar joint distraction arthrodesis, the authors advocate using 2 large cancellous fully threaded screws to maintain the distraction and position of the tricortical cancellous bone graft as well as the position of the talus relative to the calcaneus. Additionally, the 2 large fully threaded positional screws

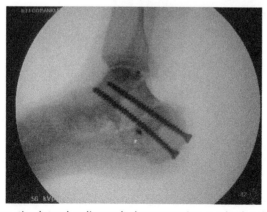

Fig. 7. An intraoperative lateral radiograph demonstrating a subtalar distraction arthrodesis realigning the hind foot and ankle. Two large fully threaded positional screws are used from inferior to superior.

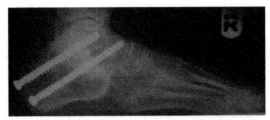

Fig. 8. A postoperative lateral radiograph following incorporation of tricortical cancellous bone graft following a subtalar distraction arthrodesis for a patient who suffered from post-traumatic arthritis of the subtalar joint and ankle joint following a calcaneal fracture.

do not cause compression across the subtalar joint and the bone graft while maintaining the desired position.

The orientation of the fixation can be inserted from the talus to the calcaneus or from the calcaneus to the talus. The authors advocate inserting the fixation from the calcaneus to the talus. The advantage of inserting the fixation from the calcaneus to the talus is that the bone in the talus is much more dense and compact than in the calcaneus, and therefore better fixation can be achieved. Another advantage is the surgeon can avoid the possible injury to the neuromuscular structures that run along the anterior talus. Last, inserting the fixation from the calcaneus to the talus allows for targeted

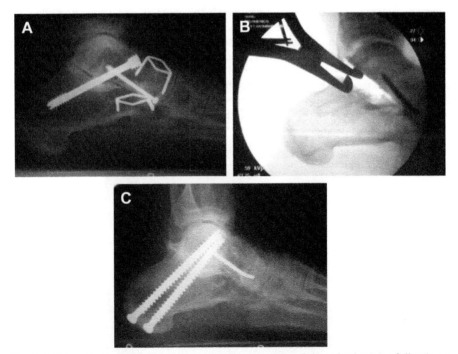

Fig. 9. (A) A patient who suffers from a painful nonunion of the subtalar joint following a triple arthrodesis. (B) An intraoperative lateral view exposing the subtalar joint in preparation for an arthrodesis. (C) A postoperative lateral view demonstrating a good bony union of the subtalar joint following revision surgery of the subtalar joint with bone graft.

areas of the talar dome as well as the talar head and neck. The authors advocate 2 large threaded cancellous screws to provide more stability and prevent rotation.

POSTOPERATIVE PROTOCOL

The patient is placed in a below-knee plaster cast for 2 weeks and then transitioned to a below-knee fiberglass cast for an additional 4 to 6 weeks. Once trabeculation is noted, the patient is transitioned to a walking boot for an additional 2 to 4 weeks. They are then transitioned to regular shoe gear as tolerated.

COMPLICATIONS

Hematoma, seroma, incision dehiscence, ulceration, and neuritis can occur postoperatively.

Soft tissue infection is managed with culture and sensitivity, antibiotics, local wound care, and surgical debridement if necessary.

As with any arthrodesis, nonunion, delayed union, and malunion are possible. Higher rates of nonunion are associated with arthrodesis following posttraumatic arthritis.[17] Good surgical technique and rigid fixation will help to decrease risk of nonunion. In cases of hypertrophic nonunion, the use of an external bone stimulator may be necessary. If an atrophic nonunion ensues, reoperation may be necessary.

Malalignment is a risk when correcting deformities. Typically, a varus alignment is not tolerated well and may require a posterior calcaneal osteotomy to correct. Valgus alignment may be treated with orthotics/bracing.

Painful retained hardware can be removed once a solid fusion is achieved at the subtalar joint.[18]

DISCUSSION

Subtalar joint arthrodesis is a procedure than can be used to treat posttraumatic arthritis, osteoarthritis, a talocalcaneal, and pes planus. It also can be added to ankle procedures as deemed necessary. The goals of the procedure are to eliminate pain, improve function, restore stability, and realign the rearfoot. The procedure is known to have high patient satisfaction with low complications while preserving motion in adjacent tarsal joints.

REFERENCES

1. Catanzariti A, Mendicino R, Saltrick K, et al. Subtalar joint arthrodesis. J Am Podiatr Med Assoc 2005;95(1):34–41.
2. Haskell A, Pfeiff C, Mann R. Subtalar joint arthrodesis using a single lag screw. Foot Ankle Int 2004;25(11):774–7.
3. Lopez R, Singh T, Banga S, et al. Subtalar joint arthrodesis. Clin Podiatr Med Surg 2012;29(1):67–75.
4. Diezi C, Favre P, Vienne P. Primary isolated subtalar arthrodesis: outcome after 2 to 5 years followup. Foot Ankle Int 2008;29(12):1195–202.
5. Rockar P. The subtalar joint: anatomy and joint motion. J Orthop Sports Phys Ther 1995;21(6):361–72.
6. Isherwood I. A radiological approach to the subtalar joint. J Bone Jt Surg 1961; 43B(3):566–74.
7. Carr J, Hansen S, Benirschke SK. Subtalar distraction bone block fusion for late complications of os calcis fractures. Foot Ankle 1998;9(2):81–6.

8. Astion D, Deland J, Otis J, et al. Motion of the hindfoot after simulated arthrodesis. J Bone Jt Surg 1997;79A(2):241–6.

9. Kulik S, Clanton T. Tarsal coalition. Foot Ankle Int 1996;17(5):286–96.

10. Schwartz J, Kihm C, Camasta C. Subtalar joint distraction arthrodesis to correct calcaneal valgus in pediatric patients with tarsal coalition: a case series. J Foot Ankle Surg 2015;54(6):1151–7.

11. Chou L, Halligan B. Treatment of severe, painful pes planovalgus deformity with hindfoot arthrodesis and wedge-shaped tricortical allograft. Foot Ankle Int 2007; 28(5):569–74.

12. DiDomenico L, Wargo-Dorsey M. Tibiotalocalcaneal arthrodesis using a femoral locking plate. J Foot Ankle Surg 2012;51:128–32.

13. Hungerer S, Eberle S, Lochner S, et al. Biomechanical evaluation of subtalar fusion: the influence of screw configuration and placement. J Foot Ankle Surg 2013;52:177–83.

14. Glanzmann M, Sanhueza-Hernandez R. Arthroscopic subtalar arthrodesis for symptomatic osteoarthritis of the hindfoot: a prospective study of 41 cases. Foot Ankle Int 2007;28(1):2–7.

15. Pollard J, Schuberth J. Posterior bone block distraction arthrodesis of subtalar joint: a review of 22 cases. J Foot Ankle Surg 2008;47(3):191–8.

16. Hersh I, Fleming J. Considerations of a midline posterior approach to the ankle and subtalar joints [Chapter 18]. Podiatry Institute; 2010.

17. Chang T. Double hindfoot arthrodesis versus triple arthrodesis for difficult hindfoot valgus deformities [Chapter 20]. Podiatry Institute; 2014.

18. Bibbo C, Anderson R, Davis WH. Complications of midfoot and hindfoot arthrodesis. Clin Orthopedics Relat Res 2001;(391):45–58.

Hindfoot Arthrodesis for the Elective and Posttraumatic Foot Deformity

John J. Stapleton, DPM[a,b,*], Thomas Zgonis, DPM[c]

KEYWORDS

- Double arthrodesis • Triple arthrodesis • Hindfoot • Pes planovalgus
- Foot deformity

KEY POINTS

- Isolated, double, or triple arthrodesis have all been studied and recommended for the treatment of elective or posttraumatic hindfoot deformities.
- Hindfoot arthrodesis can be combined with an ankle and/or midfoot procedure in order to restore the overall lower extremity alignment.
- Tendo-Achilles lengthening or gastrocnemius recession and/or tendon repairs and transfers may also be necessary to address at the time of hindfoot deformity correction and alignment.

Isolated or multiple hindfoot arthrodesis procedures have been well studied for the surgical treatment of elective, posttraumatic, and neuropathic hindfoot/ankle deformities. From isolated talonavicular or subtalar joint arthrodesis to double (talonavicular and subtalar) and triple (talonavicular, subtalar, and calcaneocuboid) arthrodesis procedures, the literature supports the impact of these procedures on the realignment and deformity correction of the lower extremity. Similarly, multiple surgical incisional approaches have been described for the double or triple arthrodesis ranging from a single medial or lateral approach to a traditional 2-incision approach for triple arthrodesis. The goal of an isolated, double, or triple arthrodesis is to restore and maintain the hindfoot alignment while minimizing any associated

Disclosure: The authors have nothing to disclose.
[a] Foot and Ankle Surgery, Lehigh Valley Hospital, 1250 South Cedar Crest Boulevard, Suite 110, Allentown, PA 18103, USA; [b] Penn State College of Medicine, 500 University Drive, Hershey, PA 17033, USA; [c] Division of Podiatric Medicine and Surgery, Department of Orthopaedics, University of Texas Health Science Center San Antonio, 7703 Floyd Curl Drive, MSC 7776, San Antonio, TX 78229, USA
* Corresponding author. Foot and Ankle Surgery, Lehigh Valley Hospital, 1250 South Cedar Crest Boulevard, Suite 110, Allentown, PA 18103.
E-mail address: jostaple@hotmail.com

Clin Podiatr Med Surg 34 (2017) 339–346
http://dx.doi.org/10.1016/j.cpm.2017.02.005
0891-8422/17/© 2017 Elsevier Inc. All rights reserved.

podiatric.theclinics.com

biomechanical forces that can result in progressive deformity and painful arthrosis to the ankle and midfoot. In certain cases, hindfoot arthrodesis and alignment can be combined with an ankle and/or midfoot arthrodesis in order to restore the overall lower extremity alignment with or without adjunctive soft tissue procedures.

Isolated talonavicular arthrodesis when indicated has been described in the literature for the correction of rigid and/or flexible pes planovalgus deformities. Camasta and colleagues,[1] in a retrospective review of 51 isolated talonavicular arthrodesis procedures to address the flexible pes planovalgus deformity, concluded that this procedure was safe and effective with a 100% radiographic union and 3.92% of delayed union rates. In another retrospective review of 26 patients by Popelka and colleagues,[2] isolated talonavicular arthrodesis provided satisfactory results in rheumatoid patients and posterior tibialis tendon dysfunction. In a cadaveric study of 8 specimens by Suckel and colleagues,[3] isolated talonavicular arthrodesis was compared with triple arthrodesis in relation to intra-articular peak pressures at the ankle and naviculocuneiform joints. The investigators concluded that triple arthrodesis led to higher peak pressures at the ankle and naviculocuneiform joints that could eventually result in their joint degeneration.[3] In another cadaveric study of 10 specimens by Thelen and colleagues,[4] isolated talonavicular arthrodesis was compared with double arthrodesis on load-dependent motion across the midtarsal joint and was found to have equal motion after arthrodesis with stability at the midtarsal and subtalar joints.[4] In contrary, Thomas and colleagues[5] have found in a cadaveric study that complete midtarsal arthrodesis was in favor when compared with an isolated talonavicular arthrodesis and the effects on the subtalar joint pressure.[5]

Similarly, isolated subtalar joint arthrodesis has been advocated for the treatment and alignment of hindfoot deformity. In 1997, Kitaoka and Patzer,[6] in a retrospective review of 21 patients, have concluded that isolated subtalar joint arthrodesis was effective in hindfoot deformity correction with minimal complications and high union rates. However, they did mention that some patients continued to have postoperative pain when preexisted adjacent joint arthrosis was evident. In another retrospective study of 95 isolated subtalar joint arthrodesis by Davies and colleagues,[7] 95% of the studied patients had complete osseous union with a single screw fixation. Joveniaux and colleagues,[8] in a retrospective review of 28 patients with in situ subtalar arthrodesis, achieved osseous union in all cases with minimal arthritic changes in adjacent joints. Yildirim and colleagues[9] have also retrospective reviewed the outcomes of an isolated subtalar arthrodesis in 31 patients showing satisfactory results when adjunct bone grafting was used for the arthrodesis procedures. The results of minimal incision surgery for isolated subtalar joint arthrodesis were also studied retrospectively in a series of 76 patients by Carranza-Bencano and colleagues.[10] Radiographic osseous union was achieved in 92% of the cases without any evidence of early wound complications.[10] However, a cadaveric study by Hutchinson and colleagues[11] has shown that subtalar joint arthrodesis seemed to significantly alter the ankle loading that could eventually lead to ankle joint pathology.

Double arthrodesis has also been recommended by many investigators for addressing the rigid pes planovalgus deformity. In 2015, Röhm and colleagues[12] have reviewed the double arthrodesis in 84 patients (96 procedures) for the treatment of rigid pes planovalgus deformity caused by posterior tibialis tendon dysfunction and concluded good clinical outcomes with nonunion being one of the most common complications. Berlet and colleagues[13] have also retrospectively reviewed 20 patients with medial double arthrodesis for correction of hindfoot valgus and concluded improvement of the hindfoot deformity and related calcaneocuboid arthrosis. In another study by DeVries and Scharer,[14] double arthrodesis (20 procedures) was compared radiographically to triple arthrodesis (20 procedures) for the correction of hindfoot deformity and concluded that the there was no statistical difference in the preoperative deformity or postoperative correction.[14] The cost and efficiency of double versus triple arthrodesis was also retrospectively reviewed in 47 patients by Galli and colleagues[15] and concluded that both cost and efficiency (operative and procedure time) were significantly higher with the triple arthrodesis procedures.

Triple arthrodesis has been the most commonly used procedure for addressing the hindfoot rigid deformity or flexible deformity in patients with morbid obesity. In a retrospective study by Frost and colleagues,[16] triple arthrodesis combined with lateral column lengthening in 27 patients concluded radiographic correction in 89.7% of their population. In another retrospective study of 30 consecutive patients by Ohly and colleagues,[17] they concluded that triple arthrodesis with allograft and a single lateral incision had 100% union rate without recurrence of deformity within 1-year follow-up. Moore and colleagues[18] have also retrospectively reviewed 70 patients with triple arthrodesis whereby a single-incision lateral approach was compared with the traditional 2-incision approach and concluded that no statistical difference was seen in the deformity correction or postoperative complications. Surgical incision approaches have been described from a single medial approach to double arthrodesis,[19,20] lateral[17,18] or medial single approach for triple arthrodesis, traditional 2-incision approach for triple arthrodesis, and most recently arthroscopic approach to double and/or triple arthrodesis.[21] In a cadaveric study of 14 randomized specimens by Phisitkul and colleagues,[22] the vascular disruption to the talus, which was determined by computed tomography angiography, compared the single medial incision versus the traditional 2-incision (medial and lateral) for triple arthrodesis. They concluded that the single medial incision consistently disrupted the vascular supply to the talar body, whereas the 2-incision approach had variable vascular disruptions to the talar head and neck.[22] In addition, the calcaneocuboid joint was not adequately prepared and accessed through the single medial incision.[22]

INDICATIONS

Posterior tibialis tendon dysfunction leads to attenuation of the spring ligament, peritalar subluxation, and subsequent pes planovalgus deformity. Conversely, peroneal tendon dysfunction may lead to lateral hindfoot/ankle instability and subsequent acquired pes cavovarus deformity. Primary, posttraumatic, and/or inflammatory arthritis may also create a rigid and painful hindfoot with or without deformity.

Primary isolated, double, or triple arthrodesis in elective reconstruction is patient dependent and may be accompanied by adjunctive procedures, such as a medial displacement calcaneal osteotomy, lateral column lengthening, tendon transfer, and/or equinus correction with tendo-Achilles lengthening or gastrocnemius recession.[23] In addition, multiple surgical incision approaches have been described in the literature with comparative outcomes for any of the double or triple arthrodesis procedures; a thorough understanding of the anatomic landmarks and access to joint preparation is crucial for the hindfoot deformity correction (**Fig. 1**).

In most cases, hindfoot posttraumatic deformities may require an isolated arthrodesis. For example, most talus and calcaneal fractures that result in posttraumatic arthritis usually require an isolated subtalar joint arthrodesis as opposed to a triple arthrodesis with consideration in some patients with a preexisted degree of arthritis at the talonavicular and calcaneocuboid joints. In contrary, posttraumatic deformities of the hindfoot that result in significant peri-talar deformity and subluxation may require double or triple arthrodesis.

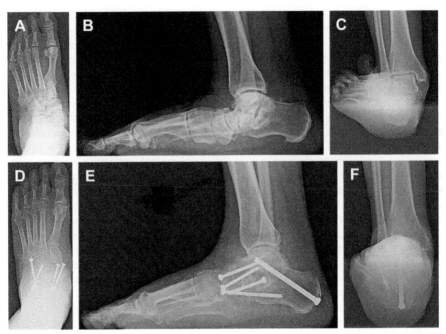

Fig. 1. Preoperative anteroposterior (*A*), lateral, (*B*) and calcaneal axial (*C*) left foot radiographic views showing a severe rigid acquired pes planovalgus deformity secondary to posterior tibialis tendon dysfunction. Patient underwent a triple arthrodesis with internal fixation and a traditional 2-incision approach with an adjunctive gastrocnemius recession. Postoperative anteroposterior (*D*), lateral (*E*), and calcaneal axial (*F*) left foot radiographic views showing anatomic alignment and osseous union at 12-month follow-up.

Hindfoot and/or ankle rheumatoid or neuropathic deformities, such as Charcot neuroarthropathy, may also warrant double, triple, ankle, tibiocalcaneal, or tibiotalocalcaneal arthrodesis based on the presence of an open wound, osteomyelitis, anatomic location, severity of deformity, ambulatory status, vascular supply, and management of medical comorbidities.

PREOPERATIVE PLANNING

A detailed history and physical examination are important in order to determine the patients' surgical procedure and proper postoperative course. Patients are examined in a non–weight bearing and standing position and during gait analysis. Tendon and muscle strength are examined for the posterior tibialis tendon with a single heel rise test, peroneal tendons, and equinus contracture. It is important to differentiate between a rigid versus flexible hindfoot deformity and also determine the presence of any underlying neuromuscular disorders and/or associated ankle deformity or instability. Often, stress radiographs of the ankle are performed to evaluate for ankle instability if necessary. The presence of equinus contracture needs to be assessed in order to determine the need for an adjunctive percutaneous tendo-Achilles lengthening or gastrocnemius recession.

Weight-bearing radiographs of the foot, ankle, calcaneal axial, and lower extremity views need to be obtained before the surgical reconstruction. Medical imaging, such as computed tomography or MRI, may also be necessary for surgical planning or in the presence of a tendon rupture. When considering an isolated, double, or triple arthrodesis, it is imperative to evaluate for an ankle and midfoot deformity and/or arthrosis as well.

Special emphasis is given to the surgical incision planning in the hindfoot posttraumatic deformities and/or revision surgeries. These patients usually present with a poor soft tissue envelope and previous scar contractures. For example, when a failed isolated talonavicular arthrodesis needs to be revised with triple arthrodesis for deformity correction and hindfoot alignment, a 2-incision approach (medial and lateral) might be necessary in order to access all hindfoot joints and correct the lateral column if needed. Lateral column lengthening is often required to obtain correction of acquired pes planovalgus deformities, and advantages of adequate joint preparation and deformity correction prevent nonunion and/or malunion with the traditional 2-incision approach. Revision cases that had a previous talonavicular nonunion are challenging to encounter because of significant bone loss and probable need for bone resection of the calcaneocuboid joint in order to reestablish alignment of both the medial and lateral columns of the foot.

Severe acquired pes planovalgus deformities commonly present with supination of the forefoot that becomes more evident after realignment of the hindfoot. Often, an adjunct isolated first tarsometatarsal arthrodesis to plantar flex the medial column is performed along with the hindfoot arthrodesis (**Fig. 2**). Another alternative is to perform a plantarflexory osteotomy through the medial column of the foot with an allograft. In addition, a peroneal brevis release may need to be performed with an absent posterior tibialis tendon to prevent further deformity of the ankle joint. Deltoid ligamentous reconstruction when needed is usually performed with a tendon allograft rerouted through the medial malleolus and anchored to the talar neck and body medially.

Severe cavovarus deformities that require a hindfoot arthrodesis have to be assessed for a posterior tibialis tendon release, lengthening, and/or transfer to eliminate the deforming force. Cavovarus deformities is more evident in patients with peroneal tendon dysfunction and/or lateral ankle instability whereby an overpowering posterior tibialis tendon can result in further deformity of an acquired ankle varus. Symptomatic ankle instability may require an adjunctive lateral ligament reconstruction with a split portion of the peroneal tendons or allograft in conjunction with a double or triple arthrodesis.

SURGICAL CONSIDERATIONS

Meticulous joint preparation cannot be overemphasized when performing an isolated, double, or triple arthrodesis for hindfoot correction. Understanding the shape and

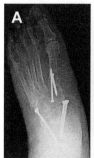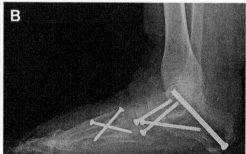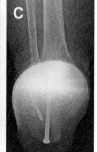

Fig. 2. Postoperative anteroposterior (*A*), lateral (*B*), and calcaneal axial (*C*) left foot radiographic views showing an adjunctive first tarsometatarsal joint arthrodesis in conjunction with a triple arthrodesis to address the hindfoot deformity with forefoot supinatus.

anatomic landmarks of all 3 joints in relation to the ankle and midfoot will ensure adequate articular cartilage resection and proper alignment. Drilling of the subchondral bone will also allow for vascular ingrowth by creating a local autogenous bone graft source to enhance the osseous union. Autogenous and/or allogenic bone grafting may also be required in certain cases of bone loss and revision surgery.

Fixation for double or triple arthrodesis may begin with the talonavicular joint followed by the subtalar joint and the calcaneocuboid joint if necessary. Proceeding in this order facilitates the deformity correction while maintaining the anatomic alignment throughout the procedure by first performing the talonavicular arthrodesis. Proper positioning of the calcaneus underneath the talus is crucial while reducing and fixating the talonavicular joint. Lateral displacement of the calcaneus can produce a hindfoot valgus with an associated deformity force and higher incidence of nonunion and malunion at the hindfoot arthrodesis sites. Equinus correction and tendon repair and/or transfer may also be necessary as adjunctive procedures.

Screw fixation seems to be advantageous compared with other forms of fixation when performing a hindfoot arthrodesis by maximizing compression and rigidity. In certain cases, such as rheumatoid arthritis, Charcot neuroarthropathy, avascular necrosis, osteopenia, significant bone loss, and/or revision surgery, the utilization of a multiplane circular external fixator may be advantageous for deformity correction and anatomic alignment (**Fig. 3**).

COMPLICATIONS

One of the most common complications of hindfoot arthrodesis is a malunion and/or nonunion. Meticulous joint preparation and cartilage resection, intraoperative deformity correction and alignment, and rigid fixation are necessary in order to minimize any potential postoperative complications. Wound dehiscence and infection are more common in patients with revision surgery, posttraumatic deformity with poor soft tissue envelope, smoking history, peripheral vascular disease, and poorly

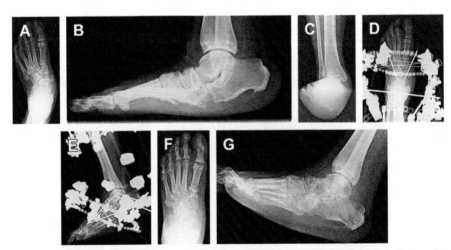

Fig. 3. Preoperative anteroposterior (*A*), lateral (*B*), and calcaneal axial (*C*) left foot radiographic views showing a hindfoot deformity as a result a Charcot neuroarthropathy. Patient underwent a triple arthrodesis with the utilization of a multiple circular external fixation device (*D*, *E*). Postoperative anteroposterior (*F*) and lateral (*G*) left foot radiographic views showing anatomic alignment and osseous union at 6-month follow-up.

controlled diabetes mellitus. Careful patient selection and medical optimization is paramount for patients' successful outcomes.

Although adjacent joint arthritis of the ankle and midfoot is common in patient with hindfoot arthrodesis, it is more evident and symptomatic in patients with preexisting arthritis to these joints. Often, patients who require surgery to address adjacent joint arthritis of the ankle are those in which malalignment of the ankle was present and progressed to further deformity and joint arthritis. Early stabilization of lateral and/or medial ankle instability at the time of hindfoot arthrodesis may prevent further deformity and arthrosis of the ankle.

SUMMARY

Hindfoot arthrodesis is a definitive procedure to address painful arthritis and/or malalignment of the hindfoot related to various pathologies. Anatomic alignment and deformity correction are necessary to provide osseous union and satisfactory postoperative results.

REFERENCES

1. Camasta CA, Menke CR, Hall PB. A review of 51 talonavicular joint arthrodeses for flexible pes valgus deformity. J Foot Ankle Surg 2010;49:113–8.
2. Popelka S, Hromádka R, Vavrík P, et al. Isolated talonavicular arthrodesis in patients with rheumatoid arthritis of the foot and tibialis posterior tendon dysfunction. BMC Musculoskelet Disord 2010;11:38.
3. Suckel A, Muller O, Herberts T, et al. Talonavicular arthrodesis or triple arthrodesis: peak pressure in the adjacent joints measured in 8 cadaver specimens. Acta Orthop 2007;78:592–7.
4. Thelen S, Rütt J, Wild M, et al. The influence of talonavicular versus double arthrodesis on load dependent motion of the midtarsal joint. Arch Orthop Trauma Surg 2010;130:47–53.
5. Thomas JL, Moeini R, Soileau R. The effects on subtalar contact and pressure following talonavicular and midtarsal joint arthrodesis. J Foot Ankle Surg 2000; 39:78–88.
6. Kitaoka HB, Patzer GL. Subtalar arthrodesis for posterior tibial tendon dysfunction and pes planus. Clin Orthop Relat Res 1997;345:187–94.
7. Davies MB, Rosenfeld PF, Stavrou P, et al. A comprehensive review of subtalar arthrodesis. Foot Ankle Int 2007;28:295–7.
8. Joveniaux P, Harisboure A, Ohl X, et al. Long-term results of in situ subtalar arthrodesis. Int Orthop 2010;34:1199–205.
9. Yildirim T, Sofu H, Çamurcu Y, et al. Isolated subtalar arthrodesis. Acta Orthop Belg 2015;81:155–60.
10. Carranza-Bencano A, Tejero-García S, Del Castillo-Blanco G, et al. Isolated subtalar arthrodesis through minimal incision surgery. Foot Ankle Int 2013;34:1117–27.
11. Hutchinson ID, Baxter JR, Gilbert S, et al. How do hindfoot fusions affect ankle biomechanics: a cadaver model. Clin Orthop Relat Res 2016;474:1008–16.
12. Röhm J, Zwicky L, Horn Lang T, et al. Mid- to long-term outcome of 96 corrective hindfoot fusions in 84 patients with rigid flatfoot deformity. Bone Joint J 2015;97B:668–74.
13. Berlet GC, Hyer CF, Scott RT, et al. Medial double arthrodesis with lateral column sparing and arthrodiastasis: a radiographic and medical record review. J Foot Ankle Surg 2015;54:441–4.

14. DeVries JG, Scharer B. Hindfoot deformity corrected with double versus triple arthrodesis: radiographic comparison. J Foot Ankle Surg 2015;54:424–7.

15. Galli MM, Scott RT, Bussewitz BW, et al. A retrospective comparison of cost and efficiency of the medial double and dual incision triple arthrodeses. Foot Ankle Spec 2014;7:32–6.

16. Frost NL, Grassbaugh JA, Baird G, et al. Triple arthrodesis with lateral column lengthening for the treatment of planovalgus deformity. J Pediatr Orthop 2011; 31:773–82.

17. Ohly NE, Cowie JG, Breusch SJ. Triple arthrodesis of the foot with allograft through a lateral incision in planovalgus deformity. Foot Ankle Surg 2016;22: 114–9.

18. Moore BE, Wingert NC, Irgit KS, et al. Single-incision lateral approach for triple arthrodesis. Foot Ankle Int 2014;35:896–902.

19. Anand P, Nunley JA, DeOrio JK. Single-incision medial approach for double arthrodesis of hindfoot in posterior tibialis tendon dysfunction. Foot Ankle Int 2013;34:338–44.

20. Weinraub GM, Schuberth JM, Lee M, et al. Isolated medial incisional approach to subtalar and talonavicular arthrodesis. J Foot Ankle Surg 2010;49:326–30.

21. Jagodzinski NA, Parsons AM, Parsons SW. Arthroscopic triple and modified double hindfoot arthrodesis. Foot Ankle Surg 2015;21:97–102.

22. Phisitkul P, Haugsdal J, Vaseenon T, et al. Vascular disruption of the talus: comparison of two approaches for triple arthrodesis. Foot Ankle Int 2013;34:568–74.

23. Stapleton JJ, Belczyk R, Zgonis T, et al. Combined medial displacement calcaneal osteotomy, subtalar joint arthrodesis, and ankle arthrodiastasis for end-stage posterior tibial tendon dysfunction. Clin Podiatr Med Surg 2009;26:325–33.

Operative Fixation Options for Elective and Diabetic Ankle Arthrodesis

Crystal L. Ramanujam, DPM, MSc[a], John J. Stapleton, DPM[b,c,*], Thomas Zgonis, DPM[d]

KEYWORDS

- Ankle arthrodesis • Internal fixation • External fixation • Surgery
- Diabetic Charcot neuroarthropathy

KEY POINTS

- Ankle arthrodesis techniques that are not destabilizing and maintain the lateral and medial malleoli are preferred when feasible.
- Crossed screw configuration for an ankle arthrodesis provides great osseous stability and compression when compared with parallel screws.
- Anatomic reduction and positioning of an ankle arthrodesis is paramount to improving functional outcomes and pain levels.
- Utilization of a multiplane circular external fixator for an ankle arthrodesis is advantageous for revision and lower extremity preservation cases.

Traditionally, ankle arthrodesis was reported using lag screws and intramedullary nails; however, with time, alternate fixation choices, such as a variety of plating techniques, have emerged leading to numerous reports in the literature. On the other hand, there are clinical scenarios that may benefit from an ankle arthrodesis with external fixation, including bone quality that cannot support internal fixation, history of infection at the arthrodesis site, and compromised soft tissue envelope. Combined internal and external fixation may also be beneficial; however, studies with longer periods of

Disclosure: The authors have nothing to disclose.
[a] Division of Podiatric Medicine and Surgery, Department of Orthopaedics, University of Texas Health Science Center San Antonio, 7703 Floyd Curl Drive, MSC 7776, San Antonio, TX 78229, USA; [b] Foot and Ankle Surgery, Lehigh Valley Hospital, 1250 South Cedar Crest Boulevard, Suite 110, Allentown, PA 18103, USA; [c] Penn State College of Medicine, 500 University Drive, Hershey, PA 17033, USA; [d] Division of Podiatric Medicine and Surgery, Department of Orthopaedics, University of Texas Health Science Center San Antonio, 7703 Floyd Curl Drive, MSC 7776, San Antonio, TX 78229, USA
* Corresponding author. Foot and Ankle Surgery, Lehigh Valley Hospital, 1250 South Cedar Crest Boulevard, Suite 110, Allentown, PA 18103.
E-mail address: jostaple@hotmail.com

Clin Podiatr Med Surg 34 (2017) 347–355
http://dx.doi.org/10.1016/j.cpm.2017.02.006
0891-8422/17/© 2017 Elsevier Inc. All rights reserved.

podiatric.theclinics.com

follow-up are lacking. Many biomechanical studies have been performed attempting to compare fixation methods; however, the results of such studies have limited application in the clinical realm, as multiple variables in real-world scenarios may affect surgical outcomes.[1-3] One of the most frequent complications of ankle arthrodesis is nonunion. A better understanding of minimizing bone resection when feasible while preserving the periarticular blood supply along with meticulous joint preparation and stable fixation can potentially improve the union rates for ankle arthrodesis. The optimal choices of fixation relies on several factors including and not limited to patients' overall medical status, presence of multiple medical comorbidities, severity of deformity, presence of infection, vascular supply, and patients' compliance with treatment modalities.

ANKLE ARTHRODESIS IN ELECTIVE AND RECONSTRUCTIVE SURGERY

Elective ankle arthrodesis can include those performed for osteoarthritis, rheumatoid arthritis, posttraumatic arthritis, paralysis, and severe ankle instability or soft tissue contracture. In 1988, Lynch and colleagues[4] studied the outcomes of 62 ankle arthrodeses for treatment of mostly osteoarthritis with an average of a 7-year follow-up. Methods included screw fixation for compression arthrodesis, transfibular arthrodesis, anterior sliding graft, and the dowel technique, with an overall 14% nonunion rate. In 1990, a retrospective case series of 26 patients for treatment of mostly posttraumatic arthritis using crossed cancellous screws in 41% showed a high overall union rate.[5] External fixation in this study also demonstrated a high union rate. In a 1994 study by Frey and colleagues[6] with an average 4-year follow-up, 33 patients underwent ankle arthrodesis using cancellous screws, yet 36% (12 patients) of these experienced nonunion. In the same study, internal compression plates were used in 17 patients, with a 35% (6 patients) rate of nonunion. Furthermore, this study found a 55% (6 out of 11 patients) nonunion rate in those patients undergoing ankle arthrodesis with external fixation. A 2002 study by Hanson and Cracchiolo[7] for tibiotalocalcaneal arthrodesis in 10 patients using a blade plate with posterior approach showed 100% union rate with an average of 37 months' follow-up.[7] This case series included patients with posttraumatic arthritis, primary degenerative arthritis, and rheumatoid arthritis and postpolio deformity. In 2005 a study by Anderson and colleagues[8] used a retrograde intramedullary nail for ankle arthrodesis in 26 patients with rheumatoid arthritis, resulting in radiographic fusion of all but one case and a high rate of patient satisfaction at a median 3 years of follow-up. A systematic review by Donnenwerth and Roukis[9] found a 24.2% nonunion rate for patients with tibiotalocalcaneal arthrodesis with retrograde compression intramedullary nail fixation for failed total ankle replacement. A study by Napiontek and Jaszczak[10] in 2015 analyzing 23 patients who underwent ankle arthrodesis for posttraumatic arthritis, osteoarthritis, and paralytic causes using screw fixation with an average follow-up of 32 months demonstrated effective arthrodesis with only one patient requiring surgical revision.[10] In a study with a mean follow-up of 4.4 years after ankle arthrodesis using triangular external fixation for posttraumatic arthrosis, Kiene and colleagues[11] reported comparable nonunion rates with internal fixation; however, they also showed increased pain and complication rates commenting that this method may best be reserved for cases of infected arthritis and soft tissue compromise. Easley and colleagues[12] analyzed the use of internal and external fixation for revision ankle arthrodesis in 45 patients with an average follow-up of 50.3 months, demonstrating that circular external fixation achieves acceptable union rates when internal fixation is contraindicated.

ANKLE ARTHRODESIS IN DIABETES MELLITUS AND INFECTION

Ankle arthrodesis for diabetic complications, such as osteomyelitis and Charcot neuroarthropathy (CN), constitute an entirely separate group that calls for different surgical approaches for successful outcomes. The medical status and multiple comorbidities in this population present with inherent complications for higher risk of complications and, therefore, should require careful consideration when contemplating an ankle arthrodesis. Medical optimization through a multidisciplinary approach is recommended before any surgical reconstruction.[13] The presence of hyperglycemia and/or peripheral neuropathy in diabetic patients has been shown to cause differences in wound and bone healing.[14] Additionally, in the previously mentioned study by Frey and colleagues,[6] diabetes mellitus was found to be a predisposing factor leading to nonunion. Furthermore, the same study demonstrated a nonunion rate of 83% in patients with history of infection. Severe instability in the presence of CN may lead to ulceration and subsequent infection; therefore, these deformities may require alternate fixation methods. Pinzur and Noonan[15] used a retrograde locked femoral nail for ankle arthrodesis in 9 patients with diabetic CN, with all patients achieving ambulatory status without new ulceration or infection at an average 32-month follow-up. Fabrin and colleagues[16] reported successful arthrodesis with external fixation for realignment of 11 patients with diabetic CN of the ankle. At a median follow-up of 48 months, all of the patients were able to ambulate with a brace; however, not all achieved osseous union. This finding highlights that the definition of a successful outcome for this population may differ from other elective or reconstructive patient groups. Acute or chronic osteomyelitis should be addressed through aggressive surgical debridement with systemic and/or local antibiotic therapy, and large soft tissue defects may be amenable to negative pressure wound therapy before attempted ankle arthrodesis.[13] Infection following trauma may also be addressed in a similar fashion. Kolker and Wilson[17] reported on successful staged debridement with total talectomy followed by tibiocalcaneal arthrodesis using interpositional autogenous cancellous bone graft and multiplanar external fixation in 3 patients with chronic talar osteomyelitis after fracture-dislocation including a mean follow-up of 31 months.

PREOPERATIVE PLANNING

Minimizing surgical complications in elective or diabetic ankle arthrodesis procedures begins with a thorough history and physical examination and detection of controllable risk factors. Medical comorbidities, such as diabetes mellitus, morbid obesity, peripheral arterial disease, peripheral neuropathy, rheumatoid arthritis, chronic steroid use, tobacco and/or alcohol abuse, and history of thromboembolic disease, must be considered in great detail with medical optimization performed before surgery.

Patients with arterial insufficiency demonstrating intermittent claudication and/or rest pain will need a vascular surgery consultation and intervention if required before surgery. In the presence of active infection and/or history of osteomyelitis, further medical imaging and staged reconstruction may need to be performed before the final definitive procedure. Radiographic evaluation of the foot, including calcaneal axial, ankle, and lower extremity alignment views, are paramount for preoperative assessment and surgical planning. Computed tomography scans are also useful to evaluate the quality of the bone, bone loss, nonunion, malunion, adjacent joint arthritis, and lower extremity deformities that may be difficult to discern from plain radiographs.

Physical examination of the entire lower extremity is vital with patients in stance position and during gait analysis. Thorough assessment of ankle, hindfoot, and tarsal joint range of motion; limb length discrepancy; and comparison of the contralateral leg is necessary. In elective patients, determining that ankle pain is originating from a purely arthritic joint is often diagnosed with therapeutic ankle injections, immobilization, or casting boots, which can further assist in the surgical decision of an ankle arthrodesis.

Assessment of the soft tissue envelope is essential to planning the surgical approach. Previous traumatic and surgical scars should be evaluated for the presence of underlying infection. Frequently, wounds that have healed secondarily or have evidence of a healed sinus tract are concerning for future wound complications. In patients with previous history of nonunion, septic joint, and/or postoperative infection, laboratory studies should be reviewed to ensure resolution of any infectious process. Often, patients with potential for latent or residual deep infection are best managed with the utilization of external fixation as opposed to internal fixation, whereas intraoperative soft tissue, bone, and histopathological cultures may be required to guide antibiotic treatment during the postoperative course.

SURGICAL CONSIDERATIONS

One of the most significant factors to consider when performing an ankle arthrodesis is the location of the surgical incision placement. Surgical approaches with fewer destabilizing techniques by preserving the periarticular blood supply to the ankle arthrodesis site, while minimizing bone resection through preservation of the lateral and medial malleoli, are usually highly considered in elective patients. These key points, when feasible to maintain, allow for improved manipulation over alignment and prevent the incidence of a malunion and/or nonunion postoperatively. However, certain clinical scenarios require resection of either the lateral and/or medial malleolus to achieve successful ankle alignment and arthrodesis. Patients with severe deformity, bone loss, revision surgery, posttraumatic arthritis with failed hardware, and CN may require bone resection of either or both malleoli in order to achieve physiologic realignment and arthrodesis.

The arthroscopic, mini-open arthrotomy and anterior ankle approach should be considered and performed with rigid internal fixation when possible, as these techniques are reliable and allow for improved union rates. In addition, these techniques allow preservation of both the lateral and medial malleoli by maintaining the periosteal blood supply, anatomic alignment of the arthrodesis site, and offer additional options if later conversion to an ankle arthroplasty is considered. Although advances to the design of ankle implants are anticipated to improve with time, preservation of both the medial and lateral malleoli when performing an ankle arthrodesis may facilitate the conversion to an ankle arthroplasty if needed.

Arthroscopic ankle arthrodesis has been reported in the literature with good and improved outcomes.[18–20] However, in many cases whereby an ankle deformity and severe arthritis is present, joint exposure and preparation can be quite challenging. The 2-incision mini-open arthrotomy allows greater exposure and facilitates the utilization of necessary instrumentation, such as sharp chisels, osteotomes, and curettes, to adequately prepare the joint surfaces. This surgical approach is favorable when an ankle arthrodesis is performed in the absence of bone loss and severe deformity (**Fig. 1**). The ankle joint surfaces can be perforated with a small osteotome or drill bit to induce vascular ingrowth and increase the surface area by creating local autogenous bone grafting facilitating the arthrodesis union. The alignment of the joint is verified under intraoperative C-arm fluoroscopy and should be anatomic in all planes. Fixation typically consists of 2 to 3 crossed cannulated 6.5-mm, 7.0-mm, and/or

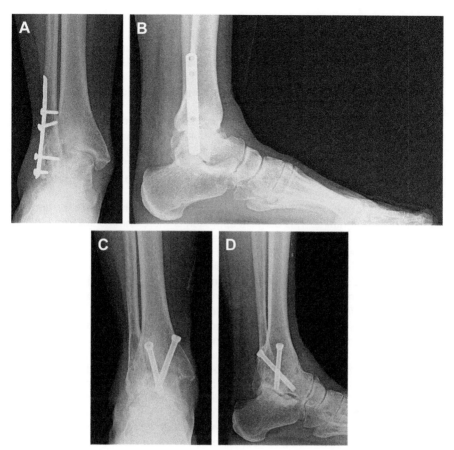

Fig. 1. Preoperative anteroposterior (*A*) and lateral (*B*) right ankle radiographic views showing a posttraumatic ankle arthritis with retained hardware and mild deformity. Patient underwent an ankle arthrodesis with a crossed screw configuration by performing a mini-arthrotomy approach and simultaneous hardware removal with additional lateral percutaneous incisions. Postoperative anteroposterior (*C*) and lateral (*D*) right ankle radiographic views showing anatomic alignment and osseous union at the 6-month follow-up.

7.3-mm screws. The first screw is placed from the posterior lateral aspect of the tibia aimed into the talar neck. The second screw is placed superior to central aspect of the medial malleolus aimed toward the sinus tarsi. A third screw is placed if any motion is appreciated after placement of the 2 screws and typically directed from the anterior aspect of the tibia into the posterior lateral aspect of the talar body. This crossed screw configuration provides improved rigidity and compression as opposed to parallel screw placement.

An anterior approach to ankle arthrodesis allows excellent joint exposure for deformity correction, facilitates bone grafting for anterior bone loss of the tibia, provides access for removal of any retained hardware in the tibia and anterior plating of an ankle arthrodesis, and also preserves both the lateral and medial malleoli. An anterior approach is performed through a midline incision over the anterior ankle. The incision starts approximately 10 cm proximal to the ankle joint and 1 cm lateral to the crest of the tibia and is extended distally to the talonavicular joint. Dissection is carried down between the interval of the tibialis anterior and extensor hallucis longus tendons. Deformity correction is typically performed by slightly altering the shape of the subchondral bone or through rotation and translation of the tibia and talus. Rigid internal is typically performed with crossed screw fixation as in the mini-arthrotomy approach. Supplemental fixation with anterior plating can be placed to provide additional osseous stability. Anterior plating is beneficial if there is anterior bone loss and bone grafting is required.

A transfibular approach for ankle arthrodesis uses a fibular osteotomy allowing for excellent exposure of the ankle joint. A transfibular approach can become a destabilizing arthrodesis technique but is used for more challenging case scenarios. Posttraumatic patients with nonunion and/or malunion, failed hardware, avascular necrosis, bone loss, severe deformity, and CN that require an ankle arthrodesis may require a transfibular approach to achieve successful joint preparation and alignment. In addition, the fibula can be morselized or used as an onlay graft for autogenous bone grafting. This surgical approach is more commonly used in lower extremity preservation surgeries that also require arthrodesis of the subtalar joint. An incision that is approximately 12 to 15 cm in length is fashioned over the posterior lateral aspect of the distal fibula; as the incision approaches the tip of the fibula, it is curved toward the fourth metatarsal base. Once the fibula is exposed, an osteotomy is typically performed about 3 to 5 cm proximal to the level of the ankle joint. The osteotomy is oblique from proximal lateral to distal medial to avoid prominence of the fibula. Patients with severe deformity, bone loss, and/or CN often require joint resection to achieve alignment and good bone apposition. The utilization of a limited medial arthrotomy to expose and prepare the medial gutter is usually required, or a limited incision over the medial malleolus is performed if resection of the medial malleolus is required to achieve deformity correction. Once the alignment is confirmed, the joints surfaces can be stabilized with guide pins for 6.5-to 7.3-mm cannulated screws and/or Steinmann pins if circular external fixation is used. Autogenous bone graft from the fibula can be used for any small defects or gaps at the arthrodesis site. When the distal fibula is used as on onlay bone graft is usually stabilized with point reduction clamps and placement of 3.5-mm or 4.0-mm small fragment screws.

ANKLE ARTHRODESIS FIXATION OPTIONS WITH EXTERNAL FIXATION

The utilization of circular external fixation for ankle arthrodesis is usually reserved for cases of revision surgery with bone loss, osteopenia, septic arthritis, history of deep infection and open wounds, severe deformity, and CN. External fixation is advantageous in these aforementioned clinical scenarios and becomes ideal in providing simultaneous compression, stabilization and off-loading for the surgical lower extremity (**Fig. 2**). Monolateral, hybrid, and simple bar-to-clamp external fixators are usually not sufficient to achieve osseous stability, deformity correction, compression and be retained on the lower extremity for approximately 3 to 4 months. A circular external fixator used for ankle arthrodesis provides a rigid construct consisted of 2 tibia rings appropriately sized to the leg and a foot plate or midfoot ring. Compression between the tibia fixation and foot plate or midfoot ring is performed with threaded rods, hinges, or adjustable struts. Smooth wire and/or half pin placement and overall anatomic alignment and positioning of the circular external fixator is paramount to patients' successful outcome, as poorly placed wires or a malaligned external fixation hardware can lead to neurovascular injury, unstable construct, pin site infections, loss of correction, nonunion, malunion, and/or amputation. Multiplane circular external fixators can

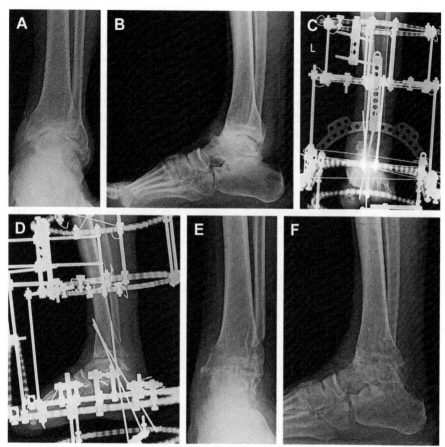

Fig. 2. Preoperative anteroposterior (*A*) and lateral (*B*) left ankle radiographic views showing a severe ankle varus deformity with end-stage osteoarthritis. Patient underwent an ankle and subtalar joint arthrodesis with a wedge resection of the ankle joint and deformity correction with a multiple circular external fixation (*C, D*). Postoperative anteroposterior (*E*) and lateral (*F*) left ankle radiographic views showing anatomic alignment and osseous union at the 6-month follow-up.

be challenging to apply and have a steep learning curve in order to avoid complications.

POSTOPERATIVE CARE

Patients who undergo an ankle arthrodesis with internal fixation are routinely placed in a bulky compression dressing with posterior and/or U-splint in the immediate postoperative period. At the first postoperative visit, the lower extremity is assessed and usually placed in a non–weight-bearing short leg cast for approximately 4 to 6 weeks with casting change intervals of 2 to 3 weeks. Patients are then usually advanced into a walking cast for an additional 4 to 6 weeks. During the postoperative visits the retained sutures and/or staples are removed and radiographs are obtained when necessary. Weight bearing is then advanced in a lower extremity walking boot and regular shoe with or without bracing over the subsequent 4 to 6 weeks as tolerated. Lack of osseous healing at approximately 6 months postoperatively typically requires a computed tomography scan to evaluate the joint and retained hardware.

Patients who undergo an ankle arthrodesis with circular external fixation may require frequent postoperative visits to assess for any broken hardware and/or wound or wire/pin tract infections. Patients with CN or peripheral neuropathy are kept non–weight bearing with the circular external fixation device during the postoperative course. The external fixators are typically removed 3 to 4 months postoperatively and followed by short leg casting for an additional 4 to 6 weeks during which weight bearing is initiated. Weight bearing is advanced in a lower extremity walking boot and regular shoes with bracing once radiographic healing is confirmed.

SUMMARY

Ankle arthrodesis remains a reliable option for the treatment of many severe conditions of the hindfoot/ankle. Although the literature has numerous short-term reports for a variety of techniques in ankle arthrodesis, this review article presents outcomes in the existing literature that includes midterm to long-term follow-up. Further long-term and prospective clinical studies should be undertaken to produce information on the efficacy of such procedures in specific populations. Surgeons should consider the risks and benefits for all possible techniques because decision-making for the most optimal approach is multifactorial.

REFERENCES

1. Thordarson DB, Markolf K, Cracchiolo A. Stability of an ankle arthrodesis fixed by cancellous-bone screws compared with that fixed by an external fixator. A biomechanical study. J Bone Joint Surg Am 1992;74:1050–5.
2. Nasson S, Shuff C, Palmer D, et al. Biomechanical comparison of ankle arthrodesis techniques: crossed screws vs. blade plate. Foot Ankle Int 2001;22:575–80.
3. Ogut T, Glisson RR, Chuckpaiwong B, et al. External ring fixation versus screw fixation for ankle arthrodesis: a biomechanical comparison. Foot Ankle Int 2009;30:353–60.
4. Lynch AF, Bourne RB, Rorabeck CH. The long-term results of ankle arthrodesis. J Bone Joint Surg Br 1988;70:113–6.
5. Aaron AD. Ankle fusion: a retrospective review. Orthopedics 1990;13:1249–54.
6. Frey C, Halikus NM, Vu-Rose T, et al. A review of ankle arthrodesis: predisposing factors to nonunion. Foot Ankle Int 1994;15:581–4.
7. Hanson TW, Cracchiolo A 3rd. The use of a 95 degree blade plate and a posterior approach to achieve tibiotalocalcaneal arthrodesis. Foot Ankle Int 2002;23:704–10.
8. Anderson T, Linder L, Rydholm U, et al. Tibio-talocalcaneal arthrodesis as a primary procedure using a retrograde intramedullary nail: a retrospective study of 26 patients with rheumatoid arthritis. Acta Orthop 2005;76:580–7.
9. Donnenwerth MP, Roukis TS. Tibio-talo-calcaneal arthrodesis with retrograde compression intramedullary nail fixation for salvage of failed total ankle replacement: a systematic review. Clin Podiatr Med Surg 2013;30:199–206.
10. Napiontek M, Jaszczak T. Ankle arthrodesis from lateral transfibular approach: analysis of treatment results of 23 feet treated by the modified Mann's technique. Eur J Orthop Surg Traumatol 2015;25:1195–9.
11. Kiene J, Schulz AP, Hillbricht S, et al. Clinical results of resection arthrodesis by triangular external fixation for posttraumatic arthrosis of the ankle joint in 89 cases. Eur J Med Res 2009;14:25–9.

12. Easley ME, Montijo HE, Wilson JB, et al. Revision tibiotalar arthrodesis. J Bone Joint Surg Am 2008;90:1212–23.
13. Stapleton JJ, Zgonis T. Concomitant osteomyelitis and avascular necrosis of the talus treated with talectomy and tibiocalcaneal arthrodesis. Clin Podiatr Med Surg 2013;30:251–6.
14. O'Connor KM, Johnson JE, McCormick JJ, et al. Clinical and operative factors related to successful revision arthrodesis in the foot and ankle. Foot Ankle Int 2016;37:809–15.
15. Pinzur MS, Noonan T. Ankle arthrodesis with a retrograde femoral nail for Charcot ankle arthropathy. Foot Ankle Int 2005;26:545–9.
16. Fabrin J, Larsen K, Holstein PE. Arthrodesis with external fixation in the unstable or misaligned Charcot ankle in patients with diabetes mellitus. Int J Low Extrem Wounds 2007;6:102–7.
17. Kolker D, Wilson MG. Tibiocalcaneal arthrodesis after total talectomy for treatment of osteomyelitis of the talus. Foot Ankle Int 2004;25:861–5.
18. Elmlund AO, Winson IG. Arthroscopic ankle arthrodesis. Foot Ankle Clin 2015;20: 71–80.
19. Kim HN, Jeon JY, Noh KC, et al. Arthroscopic ankle arthrodesis with intra-articular distraction. J Foot Ankle Surg 2014;53:515–8.
20. Townshend D, Di Silvestro M, Krause F, et al. Arthroscopic versus open ankle arthrodesis: a multicenter comparative case series. J Bone Joint Surg Am 2013;95:98–102.

Tibiotalocalcaneal Arthrodesis for Foot and Ankle Deformities

 CrossMark

Patrick R. Burns, DPM[a],*, Augusta Dunse, DPM[b]

KEYWORDS

- Tibiotalocalcaneal arthrodesis • Intramedullary nails • Subtalar joint • Ankle joint

KEY POINTS

- Primary goals of tibiotalocalcaneal arthrodesis include pain relief, deformity correction, stability, and maintenance or restoration of stable hindfoot alignment.
- Choice of both incision and fixation is based on the deformity, pathology, prior surgery and hardware, and surgeon comfort and preference.
- Intramedullary nails offer high rotational stability and limited soft tissue damage, with new constructs offering either internal, external, or combined techniques for compression.
- Peri- and postoperative fractures, malunion, nonunion, and superficial and deep infections have all been reported as potential complications of this procedure.

INTRODUCTION

Tibiotalocalcaneal (TTC) arthrodesis is a powerful tool for deformity correction in the patient with complicated rearfoot and ankle deformity. Simultaneous fusion of the ankle and subtalar joints is oftentimes the only alternative to below-the-knee amputation. Bone loss from the talus or tibial plafond, significant angular deformity, osteoporosis, the presence of osteomyelitis, poor skin or soft tissue envelope, and the presence of Charcot neuropathic joint destruction are factors that increase the complexity of these surgical techniques. An increase in the spectrum of indications, fixation options, and number of surgeons adopting these fusion methods has increased significantly in the past decade. Primary goals of TTC include pain relief, deformity correction, stability, and maintenance or restoration of stable hindfoot alignment.

The authors have nothing to disclose.

[a] Podiatric Medicine and Surgery Residency, Department of Orthopaedic Surgery, University of Pittsburgh Medical Center, University of Pittsburgh School of Medicine, 1515 Locust Street #350, Pittsburgh, PA 15219, USA; [b] PGY-2, Podiatric Medicine and Surgery Residency, University of Pittsburgh Medical Center, 1400 Locust Street, Pittsburgh, PA 15217, USA
* Corresponding author.
E-mail address: burnsp@upmc.edu

INDICATIONS AND CONTRAINDICATIONS

The spectrum of indications to perform TTC has evolved in the past decade to include patients with arthridities affecting both the ankle and the subtalar joints (including posttraumatic, degenerative, and inflammatory), neuromuscular disorders, avascular necrosis of the talus, failed ankle arthroplasty or arthrodesis, congenital deformity, instability, and Charcot neuroarthropathy.[1]

Relative contraindications for TTC include peripheral vascular disease, soft tissue compromise, regular use of tobacco products, and active infection. The presence of active bone infection is a contraindication when considering internal fixation of any kind. TTC arthrodesis in these cases can be performed after a staged protocol with external fixation and other means, until infection and wounds are cleared. Although some devices are amendable to antibiotic coats and placement of antibiotic spacers, external fixation above the level of suspected infection is justified in these cases and is discussed elsewhere in this issue. Tibial malalignment of greater than 10° in any plane is also a potential contraindication, unless corrected for, as these patients are unlikely to be biomechanically stable in the knee or hip after loss of motion in the hindfoot. Although young age is not an absolute contraindication, it should be considered. The stiffness and gait changes that can accompany this type of fusion in theory could lead to adjacent joint issues, so in younger patients this should be discussed if there are no alternatives.

ALIGNMENT

Of paramount importance to any functional fusion is restoring or maintaining correct anatomic alignment of the arthrodesis to create a plantigrade foot. The reconstruction of the severely deformed, failed arthrodesis or arthroplasty, or arthritic hindfoot is complex in that it is often a multiplanar deformity. Numerous studies define the following angles as the corrected position: neutral or slight dorsiflexion in the sagittal, neutral, or slight calcaneal valgus (approximately 0°–5°) in the frontal plane, and slight external rotation of the foot (5°–10°) in the transverse plane.[2–6] Slight limb shortening is anticipated from removal or cartilage and subsequent fusion of 2 joints, and this is also deemed acceptable.[7] Bone loss in other cases can be significant, either from the deformity itself or during correction. Bone graft may be required to fill large voids, and aid in alignment and height correction. Techniques to achieve alignment also will vary depending on choice of fixation and is to a large degree determined by the surgeon's experience with the chosen approach.

SURGICAL PLANNING: INCISION

There are several approaches to the rearfoot and ankle in terms of joint and bone preparation. Factors influencing include prior incisions, prior hardware, prior plastic or complicated skin coverage, need for bone graft, anticipated hardware, apex of deformity, bone graft needs, and need for deformity correction. Some incisions allow for access to bone graft. Some approaches give good visualization for osteotomies for deformity correction. Some approaches minimize skin compromise. The surgeon has to choose on a case-by-case basis, taking all these factors into account.

The most common incision for the TTC would be lateral, along the distal fibula, extending past the tip of the fibula to allow access to the subtalar joint (**Fig. 1**). This is a common, familiar incision for most, which gives easy access to both joints. Once the fibula is exposed, an osteotomy is performed approximately 5 cm proximal

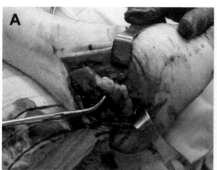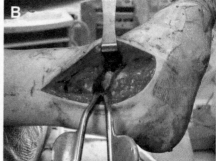

Fig. 1. Lateral incision for TTC arthrodesis showing removal of fibula (*A*) and the access to both the ankle and subtalar joints (*B*).

to the tip. This will typically preserve the perforating peroneal, which is more proximal. For many, the entire fibula is removed, to be used either as graft whole, or it can be cut in half, sagittal. The medial portion can be used as graft, whereas the lateral portion is replaced as a biologic plate (**Fig. 2**). Some leave soft tissue posterior, "open book" the fibula posterior, keeping some of the blood supply, to later lay the fibula back in place laterally. The author finds this much more tedious and uses the fibula as a good source of graft, which helps when significant deformity and deficit exist.

After the ankle joint has been prepared, the lateral incision can be used to gain access to the subtalar joint. The lateral process of the talus is easily identified once the fibula is removed, and the subtalar joint is directly inferior. This is also a useful incision if the fixation of choice is a lateral plate. The lateral calcaneus is accessible thought this incision for anatomic plates and blade style plates that have become available.

Another approach more unfamiliar is posterior. This incision is basically direct midline posterior, along the Achilles (**Fig. 3**). The Achilles can then be sacrificed, as it will have little function following the arthrodesis, or a "Z" type tenotomy can be used. The Achilles is then retracted, the joints are accessed, and the Achilles is then repaired during closure. This was popularized for select severe acute pilon type injuries as a way to access for primary fusion.[8] Although this adds surgical time, it may help fill "dead space" to minimize hematoma and postoperative complications. Either way, like the lateral approach, this incision gives access to both the ankle and subtalar. It is, however, an approach with which most are unacquainted, but does have its place. In particular, this is a good approach when the anterior skin is compromised. This is seen mostly in posttraumatic patients. During some severe ankle, talus, and pilon fractures, the skin anterior may have become compromised by fracture blisters, open injuries, prior incisions, or plastic surgery coverage, making other more traditional approaches worrisome with skin healing potentially compromised. In these patients, posterior skin is typically preserved without prior insult, making this approach appealing.

Once the Achilles is excised or retracted, the ankle and subtalar are accessed by staying just lateral to the flexor hallucis longus tendon. There is not the access to the fibula for graft as lateral, but some take autograft from the distal tibia in this area if it is not going to compromise the form of fixation. Fixation is then surgeon choice, with anatomic plates now available. A recent study by Gorman and colleagues[9] looked at the rate of osseous union and complications of 42 patients who underwent hindfoot arthrodesis with a posterior blade plate. Seventy-three percent of patients achieved osseous fusion within 6 months postoperatively, 10% experienced

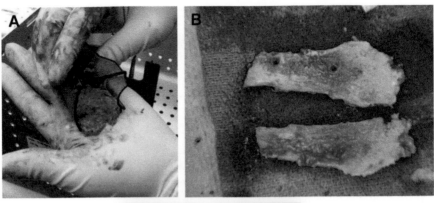

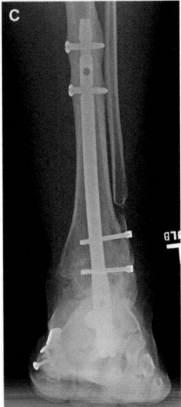

Fig. 2. Harvest of distal fibula during TTC. The fibula can be used for bone graft (*A*), or cut in half (*B*) to use the medial portion as autograft and the lateral for a biologic plate (*C*).

delayed unions between 6 and 12 months, and 18% had nonunions. Sixty-five percent of patients experienced a complication; of these, 69% represent major complications and only 31% were minor. Of note, the median number of previous surgeries in this patient population was 2. The investigators concluded that this approach had a higher complication and lower union rate than other approaches.

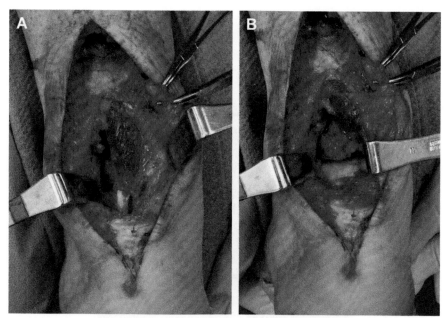

Fig. 3. Posterior approach to the ankle and subtalar joint with the Achilles excised (*A*), staying medial to the flexor hallucis longus tendon to gain access to the joint surfaces (*B*).

Most other approaches for TTC fusion are combination approaches. The options include anterior approach for ankle, with a typical subtalar incision lateral. The anterior approach is between the tibialis anterior and the extensor hallucis longus tendon (**Fig. 4**). This allows good visualization of the ankle, but obviously, the subtalar needs to be accessed another way. There is also no real bone autograft that can be harvested locally, so the surgeon needs to access graft another way, another location, or use allograft.

Another approach to consider for a select group of deformities is anterior-medial. This incision allows access to the ankle, and in some cases the subtalar joint. This approach is medial to the tibialis anterior tendon, over the medial gutter of the ankle joint and extends distal (**Fig. 5**). This is useful for severe valgus deformities. A lateral incision in a long-standing valgus deformity may have skin complications after the ankle is placed rectus. It can make closing lateral difficult and lead to tension and wound complications. By approaching valgus deformities from medial, it places the incision in an area of lesser tension to help limit skin issues.

SURGICAL PLANNING: HARDWARE

Various fixation techniques have been described to achieve arthrodesis of the TTC complex, including internal fixation (Steinman pins, cancellous screws, blade plate constructs, intramedullary nails [IMNs]), and external fixation.[10] The literature is limited and consists mostly of level IV therapeutic studies; there is no study to our knowledge that systemically compares outcomes between fixation types.

The choice of fixation is going to be based on the deformity, pathology, prior surgery and hardware, and surgeon comfort and preference. There has been a significant

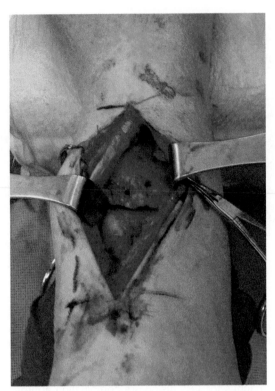

Fig. 4. Anterior ankle approach between the extensor hallucis longus and tibialis anterior tendons. Gives good access to the ankle but requires additional incisions to approach the subtalar joint.

increase in the number and design of fixation types in the past few years. Intramedullary nails, which used to be extremely limited, now come in many sizes and screw configurations, and allow for more stable fixation. Where there once were just large-fragment plates and traditional blade plates, we now have anatomic locking plates

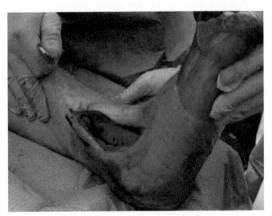

Fig. 5. Medial approach to the ankle and at times subtalar joint and medial column depending on deformity. May be useful for severe valgus deformities to limit tension on incision during closure.

for just about every approach. These improvements have allowed for expanded indications as well as improved outcomes.

The simplest but still acceptable type of fixation is just the use of large screws (**Fig. 6**). They are ubiquitous and every surgeon has a comfort level allowing their use. In the cost-conscience health care systems many practice in, this may be a viable option. One must try to orient screws in different planes and purchase cortical bone for adequate strength. Traditional screws placed from inferior calcaneus, through the talus, and into the tibia must be angled in ways to purchase the cortical bone if possible. If large screws end in the medullary metaphyseal distal tibia, there is chance of loosening and toggling (**Fig. 7**). The author's experience is that they are mainly used as adjuncts and not typically as the sole fixation.

Plates can be applied in many methods for TTC arthrodesis. The earliest plates used were just large-fragment plates or blade plates. Blade plates allow for fixed angle fixation in the calcaneus; however, the blade length is limited when applied after a lateral incision by the width of the calcaneus, typically 30 mm. This short blade placed into a mostly cancellous calcaneus does not control sagittal forces well. Blade plates also can be placed from the posterior incision into the talar neck, allowing for a longer blade, but does not include the subtalar joint, so additional fixation would be required for the arthrodesis (**Fig. 8**).

Because the lateral incision is so common, many companies have designed lateral plates, spanning both joints. Most of these plates also carry locking plate technology, which can be useful in the cancellous calcaneus and with some of the osteopenic pathology seen with certain deformities. These plates also allow for multiple screws placed in multiple planes. All these factors together in theory should improve stability and aid in better outcomes (**Fig. 9**).

Anatomic plates are now being made for anterior and posterior as well, increasing the armamentarium for those taking on these difficult patients. These new plates can fixate both joints concurrently. Many are locking technology but have variable angles to accommodate anatomy. These methods can be useful in certain deformities. In

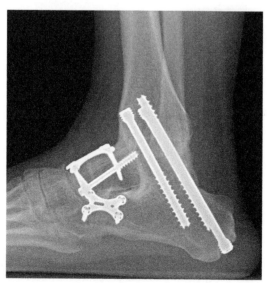

Fig. 6. TTC arthrodesis with multiple large-fragment screws purchasing cortical bone.

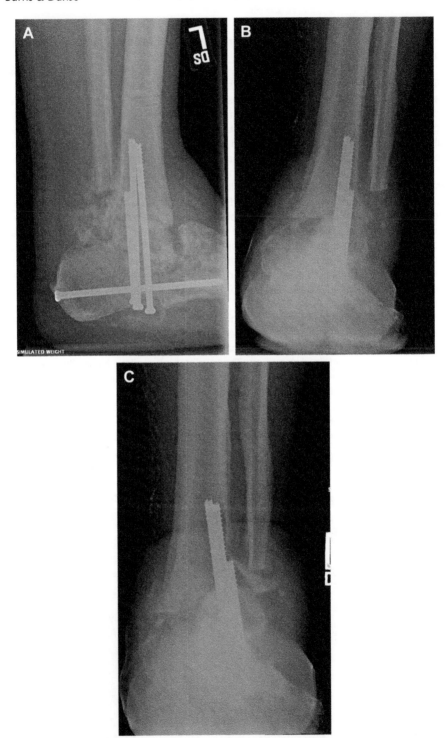

Fig. 7. TTC arthrodesis with large-fragment screws (*A*, *B*). Notice they are all similar plane and in soft metaphyseal bone, leading to loss of reduction, fracture of the distal lateral tibial cortex, and failure into valgus (*C*).

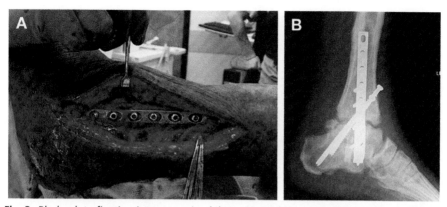

Fig. 8. Blade plate fixation intraoperative (A). Notice with time potential for failure due to soft cancellous bone and its difficulty controlling sagittal movement with lucent areas around the "blade" itself and ankle nonunion (B).

the case of revision, or depending on pathology, the anterior calcaneus can be compromised, which limits fixation with certain plates and intramedullary fixation. The tuber of the calcaneus is typically spared, making the anterior and posterior plating favorable, achieving fixation in the best available bone (**Fig. 10**). In the author's experience, the issue with anterior plating is skin coverage. Typically the anterior skin and soft tissues are thin and limited. Surgeons must be careful that any anterior plate used either has enough good soft tissue to cover without tension or choose a different form of fixation. Posterior obviously does not have this issue.

One of the most common types of fixation for TTC arthrodesis is the IMN. The initial concept of intramedullary fixation is credited to Professor Gerhard Kuntscher, a German surgeon whose use of medullary nailing remained mostly secret during World War II. It was only on return home from combat following the War's end that soldiers were discovered to have this new technology of IMNs fixating long bone fractures.

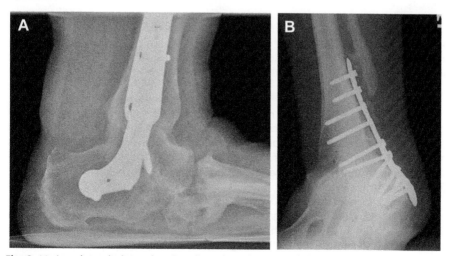

Fig. 9. Various lateral plates showing the anatomic nature (A) and variable angle locking configurations (B) that allow for improved TTC fixation.

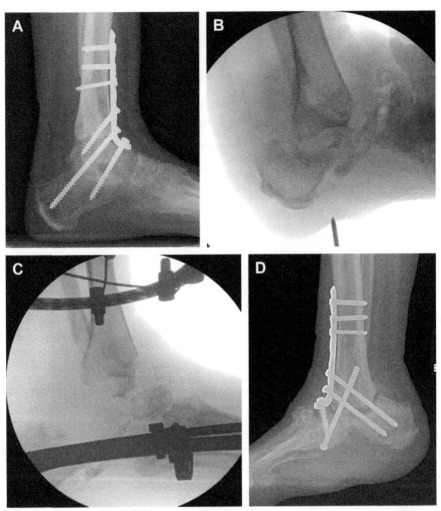

Fig. 10. Anterior plate used for TTC (*A*). This can be particularly useful when the calcaneal tuberosity is the only part of the calcaneus that still has adequate bone quality for fixation, as this patient who had staged salvage to a TTC arthrodesis after EF (*B–D*).

There are many types of IMN now available to the foot and ankle surgeon. They now vary in diameter, length, screw orientation, and ability for compression, and some have a lateral bend to correct to anatomy. The overall technique for all is similar, but it is useful for the surgeon to know the nuances (not the purpose of this article), as there may be certain times where one is preferred over another (**Fig. 11**).

The general principles for TTC with IMN start with the same TTC preparation with osteotomies as needed to prepare the joints and achieve alignment. A guide pin is then placed from inferior through the calcaneus, aimed through the lateral process of the talus, and into to tibia midline (**Fig. 12**). This can be the most difficult part of the procedure, balancing abnormal or missing anatomy, dealing with bone graft, and maintaining all these variables while driving the guide pin. Preparing with

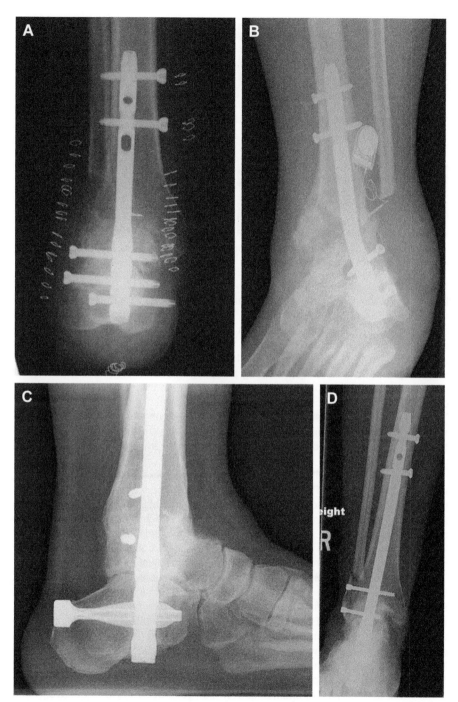

Fig. 11. Examples of IMN fixation in TTC arthrodesis. Straight IMN (*A*), bent IMN more anatomically correct (*B*), posterior blade for increased cancellous fixation (*C*), long nail to accommodate prior EF sites to limit stress on tibia (*D*).

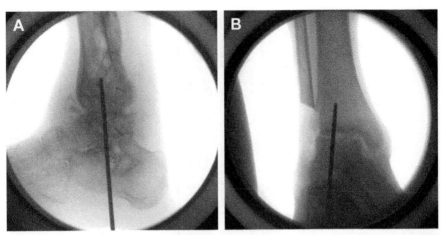

Fig. 12. Intraoperative imaging showing proper guide pin placement for IMN on lateral (*A*) and anteroposterior images (*B*).

fluoroscopy and marking certain landmarks can be useful to act as a guide for pin insertion.[7,11] Once this is achieved, the canal is opened with a large drill bit. The intramedullary canal of the tibia is then widened or reamed until the appropriate size to accommodate the IMN. Typically, the canal is reamed 1.5 sizes or millimeters above the size of the IMN selected to allow placement. If the canal is too tight, the nail will split or fracture the tibia during placement. Once the canal is reamed, the nail is placed using fluoroscopy for proper placement. The interlocking and cross-locking screws and any compression are then performed based on the IMN used. This can then be augmented with additional large cannulated screws or lateral plates if desired (**Fig. 13**). There are many other aspects that are not covered in this article, including choosing diameter and length and the biomechanics and strengths of IMN.

The main advantage of IMNs is the high primary stability that they offer, particularly against rotational forces. They also significantly reduce the sustained soft tissue damage, and in certain indications, allow for earlier return to activities than traditional plate or screw constructs. Numerous biomechanical studies have been undertaken to compare these different fixation modalities. Goebel and colleagues[12] concluded that a retrograde IMN has greater mechanical stability due to its ability to adequately maintain alignment and provide superior axial and rotational stability.

Disadvantages of an IMN include surgeon learning curve, limited compression of the fusion sites, nonunion reported as high as 57%,[13] and that all deformity must be corrected at the time of fixation, which can put stress on neurovascular bundles if not performed as part of a staged procedure. Augmentation of IMN fixation with additional fixation and bone stimulation has been studied in the literature, although to a lesser degree and without any recommendations for standardization. Early IMNs did not have the capability of internally applying compression, as they were designed to achieve compression either manually or conjunction with additional fixation. In his biomechanical examination of first-generation IMNs in cadaveric and synthetic specimens, Yakacki and colleagues[14] found that intramedullary compression forces decreased by 90% once the external compressive forces were removed. They postulated that the loss of compression could lead to instability with subsequent increased risk of hardware failure or nonunion. Newer IMNs now have internal,

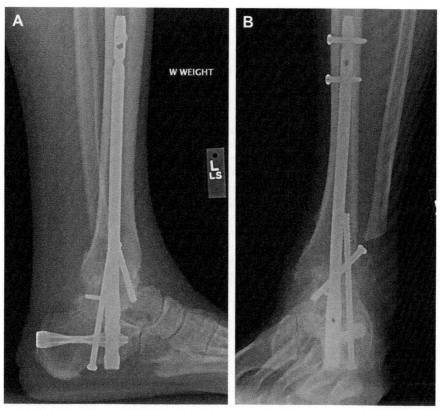

Fig. 13. Augmentation of IMN with large screws, to add stability with fixation in multiple planes (*A*, *B*).

external, or combined techniques for compression during the application of the IMN to combat this loss of stability. In biomechanical studies, systems with internal compression have demonstrated superior compressive strength to those that rely on external compression. Others supplement large screws to add compression and stability gaining fixation in multiple planes. Taylor and colleagues[15] retrospectively compared 198 IMNs with and without internal compression, and found that procedures performed without internal compression resulted in a greater proportion of nonunions at the subtalar joint (*P* = .03) and the ankle arthrodesis sites (*P* = .001). After controlling for diabetes, the difference in fusion rate between nails with and without internal compression remained significant for the ankle joint portion, but not the subtalar joint. Time to fusion at these 2 joints was also not significantly different between the different compressions when diabetes was controlled for. They attribute the trend toward superior fusion with the internally compressed nail was related to sustained compression, which decreased micromotion. DeVries and colleagues[16] compared outcomes after IMN for TTC with either internal or external electrical bone stimulation in 154 patients and found no significant difference in either union rate (81.3% and 82.5%) or clinical scores.

IMN also can be performed in conjunction with local antibiotic delivery.[17] A thin coat of polymethylmethacrylate impregnated with antibiotic can be placed on the nail before insertion (**Fig. 14**). This can be useful in patients with a history of osteo-myelitis or wounds in the area of surgery as a temporary adjunct. One must allow for the extra width by reaming to a larger diameter and must leave the original holes for cross-lock fixation open for screw placement. This technique allows for the stability of a fixed angle construct as well as serves as a conduit for temporary local antibiotic delivery.

External fixation (EF) is another option in TTC arthrodesis. This may have a few uses in particular. In patients with open wounds, this may be used as the sole fixation or may be used as a primary stage in salvage. In many patients with open wounds, or bone infection, EF can maintain position and allow for stability, which aids in soft tissue healing and infection control. Once the joints are prepared, the infected bone removed, and osteotomies made, EF can be used to maintain position until a later date, once infection has cleared. This makes any future surgery easier, as position has already been achieved. The EF also can be compressed during the infection management and may actually achieve arthrodesis in the presence of infection or a septic fusion. Advantages of EF include minimization of soft tissue damage in patients with poor skin or peripheral vascular disease, and the ability to correct malalignment both at the time or surgery and gradually during the postoperative period. Placing this technique at a disadvantage is the risk of pin tract infection, surgeon learning curve, cost, and patient compliance and tolerance issues.[13] EF is covered more thoroughly elsewhere in this issue.

POSTOPERATIVE MANAGEMENT

Patients are typically placed in a compression splint immediately after surgery and admitted for at least overnight. This allows examination of the splint and any drain the next day before discharge home. Certainly some patients stay longer or are

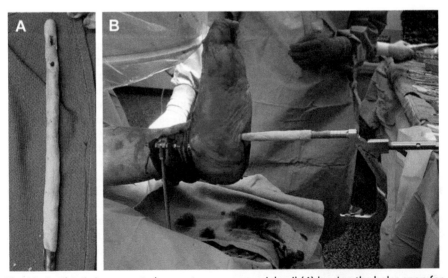

Fig. 14. Antibiotic-impregnated cement on a commercial nail (*A*) leaving the holes open for cross-locking screws. Placement of the antibiotic nail during TTC in a patient with history of wounds surrounding ankle (*B*).

discharged to a facility depending on needs. As there tends to be some drainage and blood ooze, the splint is many times changed before discharge to limit posterior heel maceration. If placed intraoperatively, the drain is removed before discharge. Many now receive a postoperative incisional negative-pressure vacuum device instead of a drain. This is initially attached to the traditional canister but switched to the disposable before discharge. The battery lasts until their first postoperative visit in 1 week. The incisional negative-pressure device aids in removing drainage but seems to aid in local tension and edema, which is useful in some of these "high-risk" incisions.

The first visit, the patient is transferred into a fiberglass cast, and stays non–weight bearing for the next 6 to 8 weeks depending on pathology and fixation. There is a slow

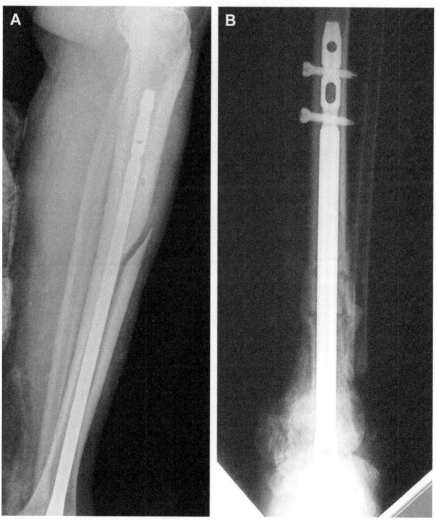

Fig. 15. Examples of fractured tibia during IMN placement with placement of longer IMN to accommodate the fusion but also span the fracture (*A, B*).

transition from that point, again depending. For neuropathic patients, the process is much longer and involves increased visits and the use of custom Charcot restraint orthotic walker–type boots for a period of months before transitioning to bracing and shoes. Many patients end with just shoes, but certainly there can be the need for continued long-term bracing or shoe accommodations depending on pathology and surgical outcome.

COMPLICATIONS

A critical part of managing postoperative complications is understanding which patients are most at risk. Although IMN provides predictable outcomes for hindfoot

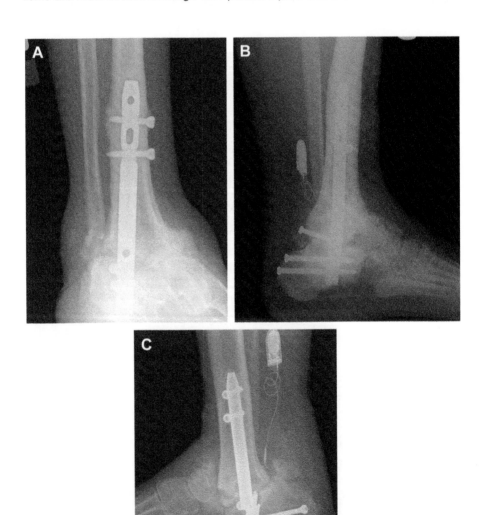

Fig. 16. Issues with IMN fixation including bone hypertrophy and windshield wiper effect of short rod in the isthmus of the tibia (*A*), bowing of tibia due to stress of fusion and short nail (*B*), and a fractured nail (*C*).

arthrodesis after trauma, it is not as reliable when applied to the patient with Charcot arthropathy and substantial comorbidities, including obesity, disease-associated osteopenia, and altered bone metabolism, and the unstable neuropathic ankle.[18]

Perioperative and postoperative fractures have been reported as a potential complication of this procedure. Fractures can occur in particular during IMN placement if not placed properly (**Fig. 15**). After surgery, successful fusion across both the ankle and subtalar joint implies a large degree of loss of motion. Without the ability to accommodate these forces at either the ankle or subtalar joint, a large bending moment can be created along the length of the tibia. An area susceptible to stress riser is located at the level of the tibia just proximal to the fixation. It is present with plating but seems more of an issue with IMN fixation. Over the years, many have realized that this stress at the proximal nail is unfortunately also at a stressful point of the tibia, the isthmus or area the metaphysis begins to narrow to the diaphysis. This junction is where many short nails end, and has been implicated in tibia stress fractures. The proximal screw hole is the most common location for fatigue fracture to occur (**Fig. 16**). A biomechanical cadaver study performed by Noonan and colleagues[18] postulated that in comparison with the standard 15-cm nail, a longer nail would shift the concentration of stress to the proximal tibia, thus avoiding the potential for fatigue fractures. From their results, they found that standard-length locked nail increased the principal strain of the posterior cortex of the tibia at the level of the proximal screw holes 5.3 times more than the locked long nail (353 and 67 microstrains, respectively). Many now use longer IMNs to gain fixation and stability higher, in the diaphysis, reducing the stress and chance of fracture.

Other complications certainly include nonunion and malunion, as well as infection. Many of the patients undergoing TTC have difficult deformities and have much comorbidity, which makes them more at risk. Trying to have the patient as prepared as possible can help with outcomes. Vascular status, sugar control, smoking, and so forth should be discussed and addressed accordingly.[19–24]

SUMMARY

TTC arthrodesis is a powerful tool for the foot and ankle surgeon. It can address many issues, and with increasing types and technologies for fixation, the indications are expanding. There are many ways to achieve access and reduction of the deformities and one must be familiar with several of these to accommodate the particular patient. Fixation is then chosen depending on these factors as well, choosing the strongest but also what can be accepted by the soft tissues, at times in combination. After surgery, the postoperative recovery is just as important to limit potential issues and need for revision. Revision of TTC will test the best foot and ankle surgeon.

EXAMPLES

A. A 28-year-old male patient with a history of a gunshot wound to the right leg, leaving him with progressive equinus (**Fig. 17**). Bracing began to fail and cause wounds to the plantar fifth metatarsal head. The wound was difficult to heal and would not remain healed with the significant deformity. He had previous grafting of the lateral ankle as part of the original injury and compartment releases, which had to be taken into account for incision planning. Because it was basically straight equinus, a TTC fusion was performed through the traditional lateral approach, but a somewhat shorter than normal incision to avoid the prior

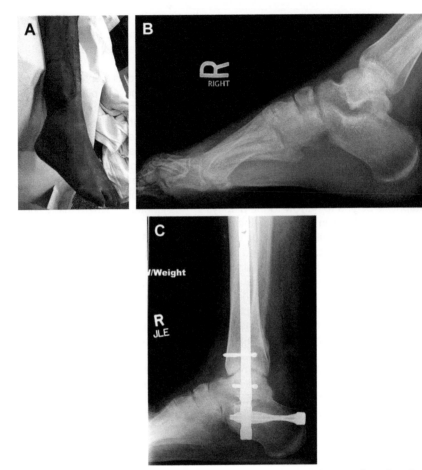

Fig. 17. Clinical picture of Example A, showing the equinus deformity, the prior plastic surgery coverage on the lateral leg, and the sub fifth metatarsal wound (*A*). Radiographs of the TTC arthrodesis before (*B*) and after showing IMN and fibular onlay biologic graft and plating (*C*).

graft site. IMN was chosen as the fixation. A much larger incision would have been required for lateral plating and the prior plastic surgery coverage would have been compromised. The fibula was used as graft and a biologic plate lateral.

B. A 59-year-old woman with a history Charcot Marie Tooth presented with continued deformity, pain, instability, and a history of wounds lateral column of the left foot. She had osteotomies and tendon transfers in the past with limited success. She had tried internal and external shoe bracing with a new wound beginning along the lateral column. She had a partial fifth-ray amputation from prior infection issues and was sent for evaluation. A TTC arthrodesis was performed from a lateral approach, using the fibula as graft and a biologic plate to gain permanent correction and offloading (**Fig. 18**). A first metatarsal dorsiflexion osteotomy was performed as well, to address the forefoot deformity.

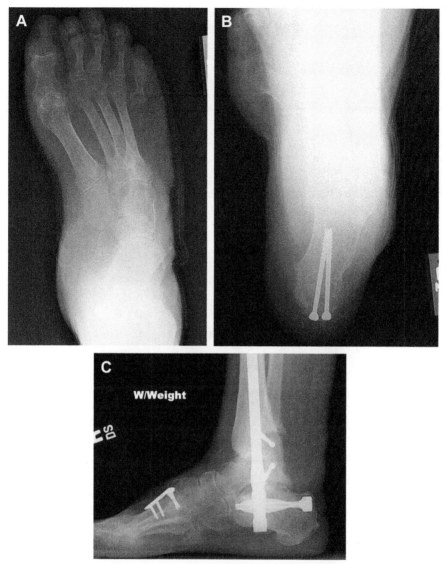

Fig. 18. Radiographs of Example B, showing the typical deformities of long-standing Charcot Marie Tooth, heel varus, and prior partial fifth-ray amputation (*A, B*). Radiograph following the TTC arthrodesis to correct the ankle and rearfoot deformity and instability along with a dorsiflexion wedge of the first metatarsal to address the forefoot (*C*).

C. A 63-year-old man with a history of diabetes, neuropathy, and a prior partial foot amputation presented with a recurring wound plantar lateral. He had wounds for the past several years, leading to a Lisfranc-level amputation. He quickly ulcerated again distal lateral secondary to the progressive equinus and varus that followed from muscle imbalance. The wound could not be healed with offloading and the TTC arthrodesis was performed in the presence of that wound. The wound was covered during surgery and the IMN was coated with antibiotic cement to help

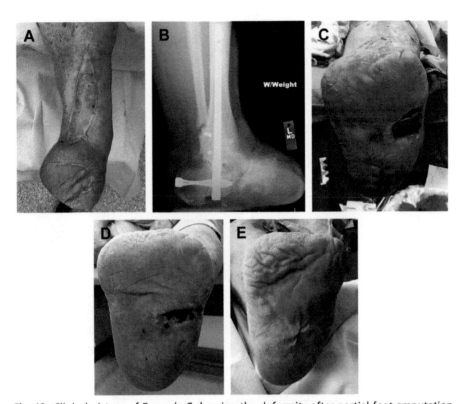

Fig. 19. Clinical picture of Example C showing the deformity after partial foot amputation along with the prior anterior ankle and leg scarring that limited approaches (*A*). The IMN used was coated in antibiotic cement before placement (*B*). Wound resolved over the next 6 weeks (*C–E*).

prevent infection issues. He had prior issues with gas infection during one of his ulcers and amputations, leaving the anterior ankle and leg without good tissue, so the surgery was performed from lateral, using the fibula as graft and a biologic plate (**Fig. 19**).

D. A 27-year-old woman with a history of tethered cord and instability presented with continued issues. She had pain and failed all bracing. She had prior fifth metatarsal fracture secondary to the instability. Years prior she had primary ligament repair but progressed to arthritic changes of the ankle and subtalar joints. She underwent TTC arthrodesis with a lateral locking plate and supplemental screw fixation to give her arthritic pain relief and stability (**Fig. 20**). The incision was lateral, removing the prior painful hardware but also giving access to fibular autograft.

E. A 62-year-old woman with a history of insulin-requiring diabetes and neuropathy presented with instability and deformity left ankle. No wounds but pre-ulcerative lateral near the malleolus. She was essentially non–weight bearing for more than a year after a fracture and sent for possible bracing options. It was clear she was going to fail bracing and had significant instability and deformity of her left ankle. Radiographs revealed a prior pilon type injury, treated conservatively secondary to her medical issues. She now had severe foot translation anterior and

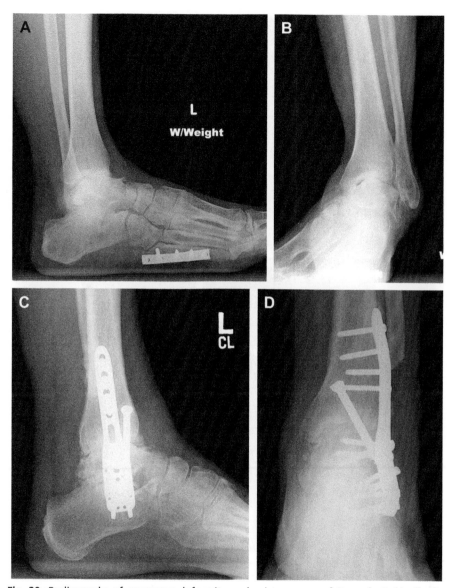

Fig. 20. Radiographs of cavovarus deformity and prior surgery of Example D (*A, B*). She was converted to a rectus, stable TTC arthrodesis with a locking plate and supplemental screw (*C, D*).

unstable valgus with a prominent lateral malleolus. After discussion, she decided to surgically address the issues. She underwent TTC arthrodesis with allograft femoral head to help accommodate the loss of height. The tibia was cut flush and the joint surfaces otherwise prepared. An IMN was used with a mostly lateral approach to the deformity (**Fig. 21**).

F. A 42-year-old man with a history of diabetes, neuropathy, chronic instability, and a long-standing wound lateral presented for evaluation. He had a large wound lateral

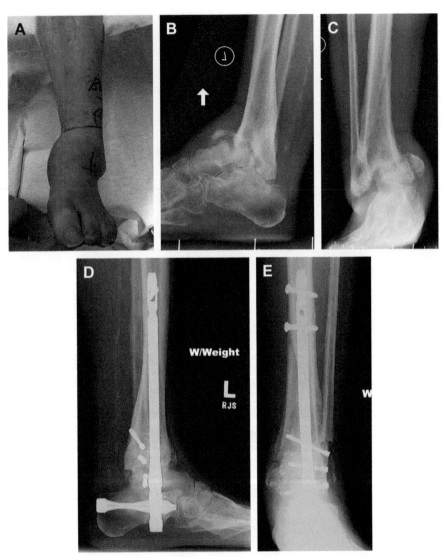

Fig. 21. Clinical and radiographic pictures of Example E, revealing the old pilon injury, Stage III Charcot, loss of height, and unstable deformity (*A–C*). TTC arthrodesis was performed with IMN fixation and femoral head autograft to aid in deformity and height correction (*D, E*). The fibula was used as a biologic plate laterally.

and plantar heel, with significant bone loss of the talus and instability. Decision was made to stage, to help clear infection, debride bone, reduce deformity, and aid in wound healing. He was placed into an external fixator with an antibiotic spacer and the appropriate consults. Approximately 3 months later, his frame was removed and he was converted to a TTC arthrodesis using an anterior approach. This permitted avoidance of the lateral and plantar skin, which had prior ulcers and now scar tissue, making an increased risk for nonhealing and infection. The anterior approach also allowed for an anterior plate for fixation into the calcaneal

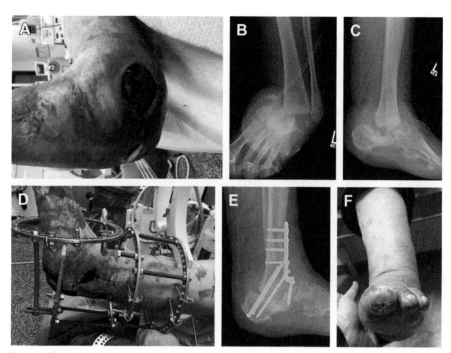

Fig. 22. Clinical and radiographic pictures of the wounds and deformity of Example F (*A–C*). He was placed in an external fixator after debridement with addition of an antibiotic spacer (*D*). After healing the wounds, and after antibiotic treatment, this was converted to a TTC arthrodesis with anterior approach and plate to avoid prior wounds and give access to the calcaneal tuberosity for fixation (*E, F*).

tuberosity, as the anterior calcaneus had been compromised by deformity and prior surgery (**Fig. 22**).

REFERENCES

1. Gross J, Belleville R, Nespola A, et al. Influencing factors of functional result and bone union in tibiotalocalcaneal arthrodesis with intramedullary locking nail: a retrospective series of 30 cases. Eur J Orthop Surg Traumatol 2013;24(4):627–33.
2. Paley D, Herzenberg JE, Tetsworth K, et al. Deformity planning for frontal and sagittal plane corrective osteotomies. Orthop Clin North Am 1994;25:425–65.
3. Lamm BM, Paley D. Deformity correction planning for hindfoot, ankle, and lower limb. Clin Podiatr Med Surg 2004;21(3):305–26.
4. Mendicino RW, Catanzariti AR, Reeves CL, et al. A systematic approach to evaluation of the rearfoot, ankle, and leg in reconstructive surgery. J Am Podiatr Med Assoc 2005;95(1):2–12.
5. Chou L, Mann RA, Yaszay B, et al. Tibiotalocalcaneal arthrodesis. Foot Ankle Int 2000;21:804–8.
6. Mendicino RW, Lamm BM, Catanzariti AR, et al. Realignment arthrodesis of the rearfoot and ankle. J Am Podiatr Med Assoc 2005;95(1):60–71.
7. Roukis TS. Determining the insertion site for retrograde intramedullary nail fixation of tibiotalocalcaneal arthrodesis: a radiographic and intraoperative anatomical landmark analysis. J Foot Ankle Surg 2006;45(4):227–34.

8. Zelle BA, Gruen GS, Espiritu M, et al. Posterior blade plate fusion: a salvage procedure in severe posttraumatic osteoarthritis of the tibiotalar joint. Oper Tech Orthop 2006;16(1):68–75.

9. Gorman TM, Beals TC, Nickisch F, et al. Hindfoot arthrodesis with the blade plate: increased risk of complications and nonunion in a complex patient population. Clin Orthop Relat Res 2016;474(10):2280–99.

10. Berend ME, Glisson RR, Nunley JA. Biomechanical comparison of intramedullary nail and crossed lag screw fixation for tibiotalocalcaneal arthrodesis. Foot Ankle Int 1997;18(10):639–43.

11. Belczyk RJ, Combs DB, Wukich DK. Technical tip: a simple method for proper placement of an intramedullary nail entry point for tibiotalocalcaneal or tibiocalcaneal arthrodesis. Foot Ankle Online J 2008;1(9):4–11.

12. Goebel M, Gerdesmeyer L, Mückley T, et al. Retrograde intramedullary nailing in tibiotalocalcaneal arthrodesis: a short-term, prospective study. J Foot Ankle Surg 2006;45(2):98–106.

13. Fragomen AT, Meyers KN, Davis N, et al. A biomechanical comparison of micromotion after ankle fusion using 2 fixation techniques: intramedullary arthrodesis nail or Ilizarov external fixator. Foot Ankle Int 2008;29(3):334–41.

14. Yakacki CM, Khalil HF, Dixon SA, et al. Compression forces of internal and external ankle fixation devices with simulated bone resorption. Foot Ankle Int 2010;31(01):76–85.

15. Taylor J, Lucas DE, Riley A, et al. Tibiotalocalcaneal arthrodesis nails: a comparison of nails with and without internal compression. Foot Ankle Int 2015;37(3):294–9.

16. Devries JG, Philbin TM, Hyer CF. Retrograde intramedullary nail arthrodesis for avascular necrosis of the talus. Foot Ankle Int 2010;31(11):965–72.

17. Woods JB, Lowery NJ, Burns PR. Permanent antibiotic impregnated intramedullary nail in diabetic limb salvage: a case report and literature review. Diabet Foot Ankle 2012;3. http://dx.doi.org/10.3402/dfa.v3i0.11908.

18. Noonan T, Pinzur M, Paxinos O, et al. Tibiotalocalcaneal arthrodesis with a retrograde intramedullary nail: a biomechanical analysis of the effect of nail length. Foot Ankle Int 2005;26:304–8.

19. Wukich DK, Crim BE, Frykberg RG, et al. Neuropathy and poorly controlled diabetes increase the rate of surgical site infection after foot and ankle surgery. J Bone Joint Surg Am 2014;96(10):832–9.

20. Wukich DK, Mallory BR, Suder NC, et al. Tibiotalocalcaneal arthrodesis using retrograde intramedullary nail fixation: comparison of patients with and without diabetes mellitus. J Foot Ankle Surg 2015;54(5):876–82.

21. Budnar VM, Hepple S, Harries WG, et al. Tibiotalocalcaneal arthrodesis with a curved, interlocking, intramedullary nail. Foot Ankle Int 2010;31(12):1085–92.

22. Didomenico LA, Groner TW. Intramedullary nail fixation for tibiotalocalcaneal arthrodesis. Int Adv Foot Ankle Surg 2012;295:453–65.

23. Lerner RK, Esterhai JL, Polomano RC, et al. Quality of life assessment of patients with posttraumatic fracture nonunion, chronic refractory osteomyelitis, and lower-extremity amputation. Clin Orthop Relat Res 1993;(295):28–36.

24. Pinzur MS, Noonan T. Ankle arthrodesis with a retrograde femoral nail for Charcot ankle arthropathy. Foot Ankle Int 2005;26:545–9.

Management of Osteomyelitis and Bone Loss in the Diabetic Charcot Foot and Ankle

Daniel J. Short, DPM[a], Thomas Zgonis, DPM[b],*

KEYWORDS

- Osteomyelitis • Bone loss • Diabetes mellitus • Charcot foot • External fixation
- Bone grafting

KEY POINTS

- Bone loss secondary to osteomyelitis in diabetic Charcot neuroarthropathy (CN) can be challenging to manage and especially in the presence of multiple medical comorbidities and poorly controlled diabetes mellitus.
- A staged approach to reconstruction is recommended with an initial surgical debridement of the infected osseous and soft tissue structures in the patient with diabetic CN with concomitant osteomyelitis.
- Surgical procedure selection, fixation methods, and bone-grafting techniques are determined on an individualized clinical case scenario and best managed by a multidisciplinary team approach with an interest in the management of the diabetic foot.

INTRODUCTION

Large osseous defects in the ankle joint due to diabetic Charcot neuroarthropathy (CN), fracture/dislocation, avascular necrosis or osteomyelitis of the talus, and/or revision surgery may need to be addressed in a single or staged reconstruction and according to the patient's past medical and surgical history, medical comorbidities, local or systemic infection, and severity of condition. Jeng and colleagues,[1] in a retrospective review of 32 patients with tibiotalocalcaneal arthrodesis and allogeneic femoral head allograft for large osseous defects of the ankle concluded that patients with diabetes mellitus were at higher risk for nonunion with an overall functional lower

Disclosure: The authors have nothing to disclose.
[a] Mid-Atlantic Permanente Medical Group, Springfield Medical Center, 6501 Loisdale Court, Springfield, VA 22150, USA; [b] Division of Podiatric Medicine and Surgery, Department of Orthopaedics, University of Texas Health Science Center San Antonio, 7703 Floyd Curl Drive, MSC 7776, San Antonio, TX 78229, USA
* Corresponding author.
E-mail address: thomaszgonis@yahoo.com

Clin Podiatr Med Surg 34 (2017) 381–387
http://dx.doi.org/10.1016/j.cpm.2017.02.008
0891-8422/17/© 2017 Elsevier Inc. All rights reserved.

podiatric.theclinics.com

extremity salvage of 71%. In addition, the treatment of osteomyelitis with bone loss in the diabetic CN has been reported in the literature with various studies and case reports. Pinzur and colleagues[2] reported on 95.7% diabetic lower extremity salvage rates on a single surgical resection of osteomyelitis, deformity correction, and utilization of circular external fixation for the management of diabetic CN and concomitant osteomyelitis. Similarly, Dalla Paola and colleagues,[3] in a retrospective study of 45 patients treated for diabetic CN foot and ankle osteomyelitis, concluded that circular external fixation and arthrodesis of the resected joint(s) osteomyelitis was an alternative option to lower extremity amputation. In another study by Dalla Paola and colleagues,[4] it was concluded that the extent, anatomic location, and stage of osteomyelitis in the diabetic CN did not affect the overall rate of diabetic lower extremity salvage. Tibiocalcaneal arthrodesis for the diabetic CN and talar body loss also has been reported by Aikawa and colleagues[5] by using a locking plate fixation.

Management of bone loss in the diabetic population with CN must be tailored to the individual and requires multiple treatment strategies and options. Bone loss secondarily to osteomyelitis in the diabetic CN can be challenging to manage and especially in the presence of multiple medical comorbidities and poorly controlled diabetes mellitus. The effect of medical comorbidities in the inpatient diabetic CN management was found to significantly impact the cost and patient's hospitalization in a study by Labovitz and colleagues.[6] In another retrospective study of 116 patients by Ramanujam and colleagues,[7] the overall lower extremity amputation and mortality rates in the reconstructed diabetic CN foot and ankle with external fixation was noted to be 6.0% and 4.3%, respectively.

PREOPERATIVE CONSIDERATIONS

Management of bone loss in the patient with diabetic CN should begin with a thorough history and physical examination by determining the anatomic location and size of the defect, joint contracture and range of motion, presence and degree of deformity, concomitant soft tissue injury, vascular supply, and the presence of infection (**Fig. 1**). Additionally, retained hardware and/or surgical complications from previous surgeries as well as the overall health status and management of medical comorbidities need to be determined and thoroughly addressed before the surgical reconstruction.

Radiographic evaluation includes foot, ankle, and calcaneal axial and lower extremity weight-bearing views when feasible. In the presence of open wounds, osteomyelitis, and/or infected hardware, advanced medical imaging is indicated. Computed tomography scans are useful for further evaluation of the anatomic region, including the quality of the remaining surrounding bone and preoperative planning. MRI and nuclear imaging are effective in evaluating the presence of concomitant soft tissue and osseous infection. Equal attention is given to the lower extremity vascular status and history of peripheral vascular disease. Basic arterial noninvasive studies are followed by vascular surgery consultation when necessary. In addition, an infectious disease consultation also may be initiated in the presence of significant bone loss due to osteomyelitis, infected hardware, and revision surgery. Medical optimization and management of uncontrolled blood glucose levels in the diabetic patient with multiple medical comorbidities and end-organ disease is crucial for the patient's healing and recovery process.

The goals of managing diabetic CN of the foot and ankle are achieving a stable and plantigrade foot that is free from ulceration and infection and allows a degree of independent ambulation. When diabetic CN is complicated by segmental bone loss due to

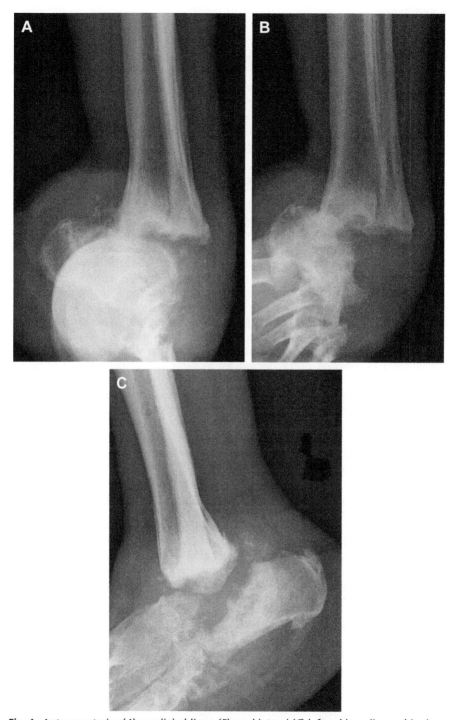

Fig. 1. Anteroposterior (*A*), medial oblique (*B*), and lateral (*C*) left ankle radiographic views showing a severe diabetic CN, varus deformity, and bone loss from a previous attempted talectomy and hindfoot/ankle arthrodesis. A thorough history and physical examination, including further medical imaging and/or bone biopsy for suspected concomitant osteomyelitis are paramount before deciding on a single versus staged reconstruction for lower extremity preservation.

osteomyelitis or avascular necrosis, the technical difficulty in achieving those goals is increased. The magnitude of reconstructive effort, patient's host tolerance, and the ultimate functional outcome needs to be considered in great detail. In certain cases, including and not limited to severe lower extremity or life-threatening infection, severe peripheral vascular disease, uncontrolled diabetes mellitus with multiple end-organ failures, and nonambulatory status, proximal leg amputation options may need to be considered as definitive surgical options.

SINGLE VERSUS STAGED RECONSTRUCTION

Currently, there are no studies comparing immediate versus delayed bone grafting in the diabetic CN with bone loss and osteomyelitis. In the absence of concomitant infection, a single-stage reconstruction might be able to achieve the desired outcome. The type of bone grafting, along with the procedure and fixation selection is dependent on the anatomic location, previous surgeries, amount of bone loss, and overall health status of the patient. In the presence of concomitant infection, a staged approach to reconstruction is recommended with an initial surgical debridement of the infected osseous and soft tissue structures. This staged approach allows the surgeon to obtain deep osseous/soft tissue cultures and pathologic specimens, as well as further evaluate for the soft tissue envelope and quality of remaining bone.

In the staged reconstructive procedures, once the initial surgical debridement and management of infection occur, temporary skeletal stabilization may need to be addressed until the definitive procedure. The use of nonbiodegradable antibiotic cement spacers and/or beads may be used for local antibiotic delivery and management of large osseous and soft tissue defects. These techniques can maintain anatomic length and also maintain stability to the surgical site until the final reconstructive procedure. Depending on the location and size of the osseous defect, application of a spanning or circular external fixation may be indicated. Parenteral or oral culture-specific antibiotic therapy is administered and followed by the infectious disease team. Subsequent removal of the implanted nonbiodegradable antibiotic cement spacers and/or beads is followed by intraoperative culture specimens before the definitive reconstructive procedure (**Fig. 2**).

The size, depth, underlying exposed structures, and location of the wound will help determine the proper procedure selection and fixation options for the definitive reconstructive procedure. Final correction of deformity and bone loss may be delayed until soft tissue coverage is achieved or may occur within a definitive soft tissue coverage procedure. In the patient with diabetic CN with concomitant osteomyelitis and bone loss, arthrodesis is the preferred method of surgical treatment for lower extremity preservation. When performing the final reconstructive procedure in the setting of bone loss, bone grafting might be necessary to maintain anatomic length, lower extremity stability, and long-term functional status. Surgical fixation options, such as internal and/or external hardware, depend on the individualized clinical case scenario, anatomic location, severity of condition, and immunocompromised host.

In the traumatic and nondiabetic patient, there are multiple treatment options for management of bone loss, including and not limited to, autogenous and allogeneic bone grafting, distraction osteogenesis, and salvage arthrodesis procedures, including shortening. Treatment options for generalized bone loss involving articular surfaces include osteochondral allograft, joint implant arthroplasty, and arthrodesis. In the diabetic neuropathic population, these options are not feasible, and bone loss is managed through correction of deformity and arthrodesis and based on the presence of concomitant infection.

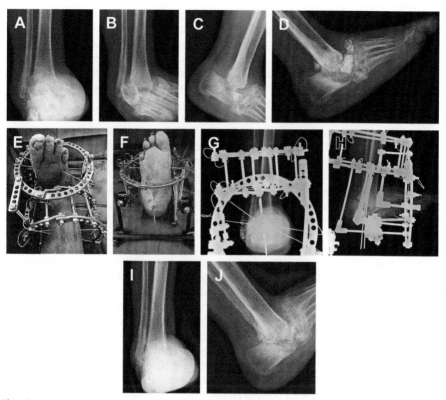

Fig. 2. Preoperative anteroposterior (*A*), medial oblique (*B*), and lateral (*C*) right ankle radiographic views showing a hindfoot/ankle deformity as a result of a diabetic CN with concomitant osteomyelitis. The patient underwent an initial surgical debridement based on the nuclear imaging results with osteomyelitis of the calcaneus, cuboid, and lateral midfoot, and deep intraoperative bone cultures confirmed the diagnosing of osteomyelitis with gram-negative rods. Two days after the initial surgery, the patient underwent a revision surgical debridement with an implantation of a nonbiodegradable antibiotic-impregnated cement spacer that consisted of gentamicin and vancomycin (*D*). The patient also was placed on a 6-week course of parenteral and oral antibiotic therapy according to infectious disease recommendations. At 7 weeks postoperative, the patient underwent removal of the nonbiodegradable antibiotic-impregnated cement spacer, further surgical debridement with intraoperative bone biopsy, and ankle arthrodesis with structural allogeneic bone graft and corticocancellous bone chips (*E–H*). Bone biopsy was negative for osteomyelitis and circular external fixation was used for lower extremity stabilization and compression of the arthrodesis procedure (*E–H*). Oral antibiotic therapy was continued according to infectious disease specialists and until removal of the external fixation device at approximately 10 weeks after the arthrodesis procedure. Postoperative anteroposterior (*I*) and lateral (*J*) right ankle radiographic views showing the arthrodesis site and structural allogeneic bone graft at approximately 6-month follow-up.

BONE-GRAFTING OPTIONS

Autogenous bone grafting remains the mainstay standard in bone graft selection due to its osteoconductive and osteoinductive growth factors and osteogenic cells.[8] The autogenous bone can be harvested from anatomic structures, such as the iliac crest, proximal tibia, medial malleolus, and fibula, among many others. The corticocancellous structure allows for cell migration, proliferation, and anatomic stability. Some of the disadvantages of harvesting autogenous bone graft, especially in the diabetic neuropathic population, are the inherent morbidity of the second surgical site, including postoperative pain and surgical complications.[9] There is also a finite amount of autograft that can be harvested from the patient that may be sometimes insufficient for the final reconstructive procedure with major bone loss.

Allogeneic bone grafting can overcome the donor site morbidity of autogenous bone grafting. The available amount of allograft is not limited compared with the autogenous bone grafting. Some of the disadvantages of allogeneic bone grafting include the lack of osteogenic properties as well as the risk of immune response and disease transmission in the immunocompromised patient. Both autogenous and allogeneic bone grafts are available as cortical, cancellous, or combined corticocancellous grafts. Selection of appropriate bone graft should be tailored to the patient-specific need and based on the severity and anatomic location of the osseous defect. For large osseous defects in the hindfoot, allograft femoral head is commonly used.[1,10–14]

Demineralized bone matrix (DBM) is human cortical and cancellous allograft subjected to decalcification. This procedure preserves collagen and noncollagenous proteins, including growth factors.[15] Disadvantages of DBM include the risk of immune response and disease transmission. Additionally, DBM lacks structural support and is often combined with a structural bone graft rather than used alone as a bone graft substitute. In addition, there are a variety of other calcium-based bone graft substitutes, including hydroxyapatite and tricalcium phosphate, as well as composite materials and resins.[16] Similarly, these bone graft substitutes are usually used in combination with structural autogenous and allogeneic bone grafts that can provide stability and anatomic alignment to the surgical site.

There are several options for bone graft augmentation of arthrodesis sites available; most focus on the use of osteogenic cells or osteoinductive growth factors. The main source of osteogenic cells is mesenchymal stem cells found in bone marrow. Bone marrow aspirate (BMA) can be centrifuged to separate the marrow cells from plasma, decreasing the volume of the injectable material.[17,18] The BMA is then combined with the structural autogenous or allogeneic bone graft to augment the arthrodesis site. The most extensively studied and widely used osteoinductive factors for the treatment of bone defects are bone morphogenetic proteins (BMPs). BMPs are members of the transforming growth factor-beta superfamily and include 18 known proteins, with BMP-2, BMP-4, BMP-6, BMP-7, and BMP-9 having osteoinductive potential.[7]

SUMMARY

The surgical management of diabetic CN with concomitant osteomyelitis and bone loss is a challenging surgical entity and successful outcomes are dependent on multiple factors, including the patient's management of medical comorbidities and severity of concomitant infection. The procedure selection, fixation methods, and bone-grafting techniques also are determined on an individualized clinical case scenario and best managed by a multidisciplinary team approach with an interest in the medical and surgical management of the diabetic foot.

REFERENCES

1. Jeng CL, Campbell JT, Tang EY, et al. Tibiotalocalcaneal arthrodesis with bulk femoral head allograft for salvage of large defects in the ankle. Foot Ankle Int 2013;34:1256–66.

2. Pinzur MS, Gil J, Belmares J. Treatment of osteomyelitis in Charcot foot with single-stage resection of infection, correction of deformity, and maintenance with ring fixation. Foot Ankle Int 2012;33:1069–74.

3. Dalla Paola L, Brocco E, Ceccacci T, et al. Limb salvage in Charcot foot and ankle osteomyelitis: combined use single stage/double stage of arthrodesis and external fixation. Foot Ankle Int 2009;30:1065–70.

4. Dalla Paola L, Carone A, Baglioni M, et al. Extension and grading of osteomyelitis are not related to limb salvage in Charcot neuropathic osteoarthropathy: a cohort prospective study. J Diabetes Complications 2016;30:608–12.

5. Aikawa T, Watanabe K, Matsubara H, et al. Tibiocalcaneal fusion for Charcot ankle with severe talar body loss: case report and a review of the surgical literature. J Foot Ankle Surg 2016;55:247–51.

6. Labovitz JM, Shofler DW, Ragothaman KK. The impact of comorbidities on inpatient Charcot neuroarthropathy cost and utilization. J Diabetes Complications 2016;30:710–5.

7. Ramanujam CL, Han D, Zgonis T. Lower extremity amputation and mortality rates in the reconstructed diabetic Charcot foot and ankle with external fixation: data analysis of 116 patients. Foot Ankle Spec 2016;9:113–26.

8. Pneumaticos SG, Triantafyllopoulos GK, Basdra EK, et al. Segmental bone defects: from cellular and molecular pathways to the development of novel biological treatments. J Cell Mol Med 2010;14:2561–9.

9. Baumhauer J, Pinzur MS, Donahue R, et al. Site selection and pain outcome after autologous bone graft harvest. Foot Ankle Int 2014;35:104–7.

10. Bussewitz B, DeVries JG, Dujela M, et al. Retrograde intramedullary nail with femoral head allograft for large deficit tibiotalocalcaneal arthrodesis. Foot Ankle Int 2014;35:706–11.

11. Klos K, Lange A, Matziolis G, et al. Tibiocalcaneal arthrodesis with retrograde nails. Description of a hindfoot procedure after massive talus destruction. Orthopade 2013;42:364–6, 368–70.

12. Chiang CC, Tzeng YH, Lin CF, et al. Subtalar distraction arthrodesis using fresh-frozen allogeneic femoral head augmented with local autograft. Foot Ankle Int 2013;34:550–6.

13. Rigby RB, Cottom JM. Lateral simultaneous reaming technique with femoral head allograft implantation for tibiocalcaneal arthrodesis: a case report. Foot Ankle Spec 2013;6:45–9.

14. Cuttica DJ, Hyer CF. Femoral head allograft for tibiotalocalcaneal fusion using a cup and cone reamer technique. J Foot Ankle Surg 2011;50:126–9.

15. Lewandrowski KU, Venugopalan V, Tomford WW, et al. Kinetics of cortical bone demineralization: controlled demineralization–a new method for modifying cortical bone allografts. J Biomed Mater Res 1996;31:365–72.

16. Campana V, Milano G, Pagano E, et al. Bone substitutes in orthopaedic surgery: from basic science to clinical practice. J Mater Sci Mater Med 2014;25:2445–61.

17. Perry CR. Bone repair techniques, bone graft, and bone graft substitutes. Clin Orthop 1999;360:71–86.

18. Bruder SP, Neelam J, Haynesworth SE. Growth kinetics, self-renewal, and the osteogenic potential of purified human mesenchymal stem cells during extensive subcultivation and following cryopreservation. J Cell Biol 1997;64:278–94.

Soft Tissue Coverage After Revisional Foot and Ankle Surgery

Geoffrey G. Hallock, MD

KEYWORDS

- Revisional foot and ankle surgery • Local flaps • Free flaps • Perforator flap
- Microsurgical tissue transfer

KEY POINTS

- Revisional foot and ankle surgery should be considered a traumatic injury.
- Limb salvage should always be the goal following a complication of revisional foot and ankle surgery.
- The approach to wound management after failure of adequate skin healing following revisional surgery does not differ from treating the traumatic injury, starting with a proper assessment, debridement as indicated, then wound closure using the best method.
- Many local flaps can solve the dilemma of wound closure for the foot and ankle without the need for complex microvascular surgery; but when needed, a free flap may still be the preferred option.
- A multidisciplinary approach with cooperation between a podiatrist and a plastic surgeon competent with all varieties of flaps could be called the "podiatriplastic" approach to best serve these patients.

INTRODUCTION

Those familiar with the traditional wound center in the United States already know and completely understand why most patients treated there typically have chronic wounds primarily of the foot and ankle. This fact is a direct consequence of their other comorbidities, including peripheral vascular disease, diabetes mellitus, or plantar neuropathy of whatever source, to list the major offenders. These can be extremely frustrating problems, as, for example, the Georgetown group has shown that a diabetic patient with a Charcot foot and concomitant skin ulcer even in their skilled hands was found to be 12 to 13 times more likely ultimately to have some form of amputation.[1]

Financial Disclosure: None.

Division of Plastic Surgery, Sacred Heart Hospital, The Lehigh Valley Hospital, 1230 South Cedar Crest Boulevard, Suite 306, Allentown, PA 18103, USA

E-mail address: gghallock@hotmail.com

Clin Podiatr Med Surg 34 (2017) 389–398

http://dx.doi.org/10.1016/j.cpm.2017.02.009

0891-8422/17/© 2017 Elsevier Inc. All rights reserved.

podiatric.theclinics.com

If the origin of a skin wound were the sequela of some form of surgical intervention in the previously intact foot and ankle, such as insertion of a prosthetic device or arthrodesis as thoroughly discussed elsewhere in this issue, the eventual outcome must always be favorable, as these differ in that they are acute wounds. They can be considered similar to but not as encompassing as those encountered in the usual traumatic "mangled foot," yet should be approached in an identical stepwise fashion to better ensure success.[2] A major difference that deserves emphasis is that management of skin complications following any form of revisional foot and ankle surgery, if early enough, can often be solved if a flap is needed by using local tissues only. Such involvement could thereby avoid the need for a free flap, and the more complex risks of microsurgery.

APPROACH
Assessment

A proactive approach by the operative surgeon to recognize as soon as possible that there is or there will potentially be a wound-healing issue will always lead to the best possible outcome. The onus on the surgeon is that for this group of patients requiring revisional surgery, it must be assumed that limb salvage is always imperative, and all steps to achieve that must be followed. Therefore, first a complete vascular evaluation to ensure adequate distal circulation is imperative, and perhaps mandatory in patients at obvious risk even before the initial revision surgery. Underlying bone and joint abnormalities requiring correction must be evaluated via appropriate imaging techniques. The presence of sensibility and perhaps even lack of plantar sensibility should be determined. The extent and location of any soft tissue deficit should be mapped by using the subunit principle as emphasized by the Duke group (**Fig. 1**), as different regions of the foot and ankle will require different tissue solutions (**Table 1**).[3]

Timing

Once a wound problem exists, and especially if bone, joint, tendon, or prosthesis are exposed, many consider closure as rapidly as practical, even within 72 hours, as the best way to prevent infectious complications.[3] Others suggest that the use of negative-pressure wound-therapy devices can extend this safe period before definitive intervention is needed.[4] Note that information available for retained total knee replacements that have become exposed suggest that in the long term even with early flap closure and chronic antibiotic suppression, half the prostheses are ultimately lost.[5] However, even for these patients, the quality of life with a functional knee was always better than after arthrodesis or amputation. The same conclusions could be extrapolated for similar foot and ankle scenarios, although there is less documentation in the literature to confirm this.[6]

Debridement

Just as when dealing with the traumatic "mangled extremity," it is imperative that all devitalized tissue ultimately be removed even if structurally of some importance. Only a pristine wound that will be closed will avoid the risk of later infection and flap breakdown. Simply said, there are 3 things that will accomplish this task: debridement, then more debridement, and finally even more debridement.[2,3] To assume that the ubiquitous negative-pressure wound-therapy devices by themselves will achieve this goal is erroneous,[7] as there is never any substitute for the skill of the surgeon.

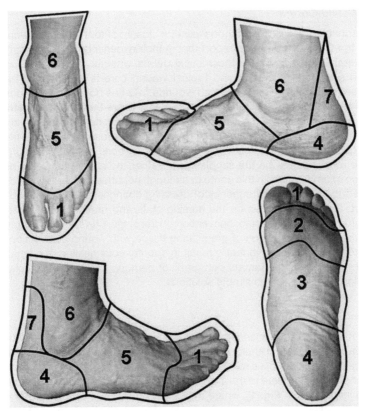

Fig. 1. Subunits of the foot and ankle based on distinct functional and aesthetic zones (1, toes; 2, plantar forefoot; 3, plantar midfoot; 4, plantar hindfoot; 5, dorsum of foot; 6, ankle joint and vicinity, encompassing medial and lateral malleoli; 7, posterior hindfoot). (*Adapted from* Hallock GG. The mangled foot and ankle: soft tissue salvage techniques. Clin Podiatr Med Surg 2014;31:565–76; with permission.)

Table 1				
Flap attributes desirable for foot and ankle subunit soft tissue coverage				
		Requirements		
Zone	Subunit	Functional	Bulk	Aesthetics
1	Toes	None	Thin	Visible
2	Plantar forefoot	High demand: push-off point	Thin and durable	Minimal visibility
3	Plantar midfoot	None	Thin	Hidden
4	Plantar hindfoot	High demand: weight bearing	Bulky and durable	Hidden
5	Dorsal foot	None	Thin	Highly visible
6	Ankle	Moderate: to allow motion	Thin and pliable	Some visibility
7	Posterior hindfoot	None	Thin	Some visibility

Adapted from Hallock GG. The mangled foot and ankle: soft tissue salvage techniques. Clin Podiatr Med Surg 2014;31:565–76; with permission.

Nonflap Wound Closure

Many reasonable and reliable methods exist for closure of foot and ankle wounds. For example, the Georgetown group report that in their experience with Charcot neuropathy that stabilization of the biomechanical defect whether of bone and/or tendon origin with adequate offloading and topical wound care is sufficient to heal most concomitant superficial and noninfected wounds.[1] As one goes up the reconstructive ladder (or reconstructive elevator, as some prefer who are thereby not constrained by climbing successive rungs in order[8]), from secondary contraction to secondary closure, then skin graft, and finally a flap with the microsurgical tissue transfer at the pinnacle; one must remember following complications of revisional surgery that the choice must not just be the simplest, but rather the choice that best preserves the function of ambulation. In this context, although negative-pressure wound-therapy devices reduce the needed frequency of dressing changes and will minimize patient discomfort, lessen the burden on the nursing staff, and prevent wound desiccation that is common with neglected conventional dressings,[4] its modus operandi is to enhance the gradual formation of granulation tissue with wound contraction by secondary intention. This can eventually result in spontaneous healing of a small defect, or allow the use of an autogenous skin graft[9] or perhaps a bilaminar acellular dermal regeneration template[10,11] as simple solutions.

Flap Wound Closure

However, if timing is of the essence, after adequate debridement with the usual use of the subatmospheric wound-therapy devices, the goal must be to use the latter only for the short term in an adjunctive role that bridges to the utilization of a vascularized flap. Any flap choice must adhere to the subunit principle according to the region of the foot and ankle involved (see **Fig. 1**), where bulk must not impede proper fit of shoes, nor interfere with efficient ambulation, while also being aesthetically acceptable for the given region (see **Table 1**).[3]

For practical purposes, there really are only 2 types of soft tissue flaps with minor variations of the theme. These can be either muscle or fasciocutaneous flaps, and each has its attributes as well as liabilities that must be appreciated.[12,13] Any muscle chosen as a flap must be relatively expendable, readily accessible, and provide adequate surface area. The major advantage of a muscle is its malleability, which is preferential for filling deep caverns, while still capable of wrapping around the 3-dimensional contours of the foot and ankle to synchronously reach multiple subunits if required. Primary closure of its donor site leaves a linear scar that is usually acceptable. However, a skin graft eventually has to be placed on any muscle flap, which may be an aesthetic detriment.

The other major option today is the perforator flap, which has become the workhorse subtype of the fasciocutaneous flap.[14] These can be constructed of any or all tissue components found from the deep fascia to the integument, for example, as fascial, adipofascial, or composite flaps.[15] The name perforator means their vascular source has perforated the deep fascia before supplying the flap. Many of these vessels in their subfascial course have passed through muscle that may require an intramuscular dissection to lengthen their pedicle. Yet the muscle never needs to be included, so function preservation will by definition be maximized. Any perforator anywhere in the body can be chosen along with its surrounding cutaneous territory specifically to meet the qualities of the foot and ankle subunits that need replacement.[16] Perforator flaps are superior for covering flatter surfaces, and usually provide an aesthetic result superior to a muscle flap. Yet depending on their thickness, these may be difficult to bend around spatial irregularities. Excessive bulk, as inherent in morbidly obese individuals, may impede use of conventional shoewear (**Fig. 2**), while making flap dissection an unreasonable chore for the surgeon as well.

Local flap alternatives

A local flap is vascularized tissue taken from nearby the defect that is to be reconstructed. Most intrinsic muscles of the foot that would qualify as such are either attenuated, atrophic, or just too small to meet the typical demands of revisional surgery wounds.[17] The distal-based soleus muscle from the leg will be reliable only if a distal nutritive branch from the posterior tibial artery exists, as the tibial head of the muscle is the longer and best able to reach the ankle.[18] Any cutaneous island flaps from the foot, like the dorsalis pedis or medial plantar flap, or reversed flow flaps from the leg incorporating the anterior tibial or posterior tibial or peroneal arteries, may sacrifice an important vascular source vessel in a population eventually at risk for peripheral vascular disease.[18] These also compromise the donor site with inevitable lengthy scars or delayed wound healing.[18]

Small defects can better rely on skin flaps adjacent to the defect if an adequate perforator still remains. There are 3 major subtypes available.[19] The first are proximal or distal-based peninsular flaps like the lateral calcaneal or supramalleolar flaps[18] that rotate about a static pedicle at their base, and often do not even require identification of the perforator (**Fig. 3**).[20] Next are advancement/rotation flaps (**Fig. 4**), such as a V-Y flap or its latest modification, the keystone flap.[21] Last is the propeller flap that has 2 cutaneous blades connected to a central hub that is its vascular supply.[22,23] Usually the latter is a perforator about which the flap can be rotated up to 180°, and can allow transfer of more proximal tissues to reach the given wound, as is commonly done today with the distal sural flap,[24] in which calf integument can reach the ankle or even the foot (**Fig. 5**).

Free flap alternatives

A free flap is a vascularized tissue transfer that temporarily is not attached to the body in any way. After harvest, this then requires reestablishment of the pertinent vascular supply to recipient vessels near the defect by using microvascular techniques to join an arterial source for inflow and a vein for outflow. A free flap can be selected from any part of the body to have the requisite characteristics needed, such as a surface area to close any size defect, or bulk to fill the depth of any wound. The choice will vary to best

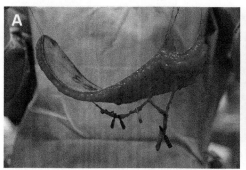
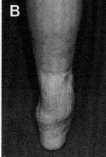

Fig. 2. (*A*) Large anterolateral thigh perforator free flap designed to wrap around the posterior ankle from medial to lateral malleolus. (*B*) Although providing a superior aesthetic result, as the flap can barely be seen in the posterior hindfoot view, even after 2 debulking surgeries, prominent bulging of the flap is still apparent.

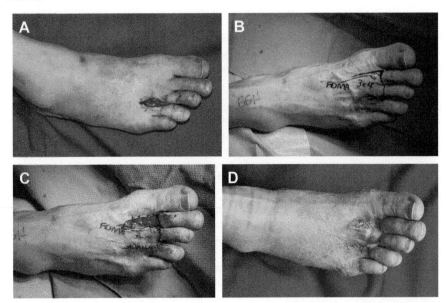

Fig. 3. (*A*) Fourth toe extensor tendon and bone exposed after adequate debridement subsequent to a wound dehiscence twice after attempted direct closure following neuroma excision. (*B*) Proximal-based rectangular dorsal foot peninsular flap originally designed on the first dorsal metatarsal artery, but altered instead on elevation to include only a large third dorsal metatarsal artery found fortuitously on the undersurface of the flap. (*C*) Flap inset over the defect, with open area of donor site medially, which required skin graft. (*D*) Healed foot.

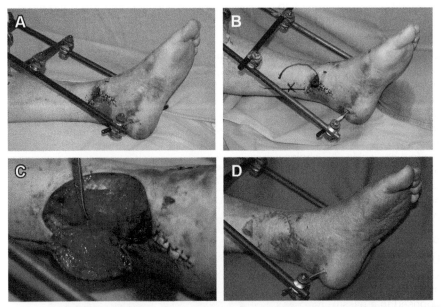

Fig. 4. (*A*) Following conversion of left medial malleolar fracture to external fixation, small area of bone remained exposed in open wound. (*B*) Advancement/rotation flap designed proximal to this wound with posterior tibial perforator "x" marked as identified by audible Doppler. (*C*) Perforator present at base of flap as predicted as shown by tip of hemostat, making this a perforator-plus flap. (*D*) After advancement of flap distally, a skin graft was needed at donor site proximally to achieve a healed wound.

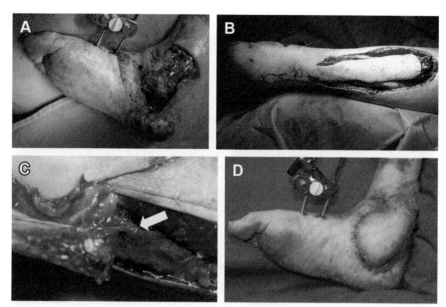

Fig. 5. (*A*) Open medial malleolar wound following debridement of delayed skin necrosis after previous open fracture fixation. (*B*) Distal-based sural flap raised with distal base left intact. (*C*) Peroneal artery perforator (*arrow*) about which this propeller-peninsular flap hybrid was rotated 180°. (*D*) Final result.

fit the requirements according to the involved foot and ankle subunit, as championed by the Duke group.[3]

The gracilis muscle for smaller defects and the latissimus dorsi muscle (**Fig. 6**) for large areas are reasonable workhorse flaps. Both will atrophy or thin in time. However, both must be skin grafted, which can be an aesthetic detriment. This is one advantage of perforator flaps that can be taken from almost any body region with characteristics similar to the subunit involved if there is an adequate perforator present. For example, the medial sural artery perforator (MSAP) flap from the calf can be relatively thin to fit the foot even in the obese individual (**Fig. 7**).[25] The MSAP skin flap territory corresponds to that of the medial gastrocnemius muscle. Because this donor site is near the foot and ankle, this choice will limit all iatrogenic morbidity to the ipsilateral lower extremity,[26,27] an important consideration. In general, a large perforator flap will often require a skin graft to close the donor site, and even direct closure will leave a vertical scar that, if on the lower extremity, also may be visible and unacceptable, which is particularly true for women (see **Fig. 7**).

Discussion

Untoward wound-healing events are inevitable following any surgery, including revisional foot and ankle procedures. A proactive attitude encourages a prompt proper assessment and treatment course that will best ensure the desired healing, as opposed to a passive reactive response manifested only once a problem is obvious that could delay the initiation of active intervention that may make further complications irrevocable.[5] Often, relatively simple nonsurgical methods can be sufficient solutions. However, experience should dictate when a vascularized flap is preferential, especially for timely wound closure, or at least a consultation for another opinion if there is any uncertainty.

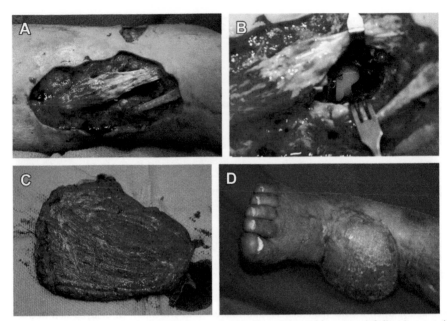

Fig. 6. (*A*) Following initial debridement of extensive right ankle wound following total ankle arthroplasty, (*B*) then retracted anterior tibial and extrinsic extensor tendons, showing exposed ankle prosthesis. (*C*) Latissimus dorsi muscle free flap selected as malleable enough to fill cavity about ankle prosthesis, while also covering entire large skin wound. (*D*) Early appearance of still bulky skin grafted muscle flap.

Any flap will add an inherent morbidity to a situation already compromised more than had been planned. Therefore, the benefit of a flap must always outweigh any risks necessary for its utilization. Local flaps near the defect always provide similar tissues, perhaps a better overall aesthetic result, may be easier to dissect and transfer, and usually do not require microsurgery and the risks thereof, including total failure. Yet

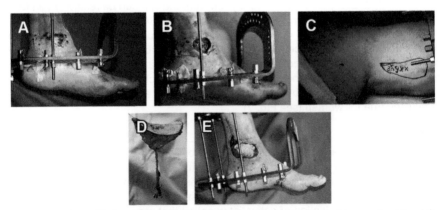

Fig. 7. (*A*) Eschar of left medial malleolus following Charcot foot revision and external fixation. (*B*) Exposed bone after debridement. (*C*) MSAP flap designed on ipsilateral calf just above external fixator. (*D*) Lengthy single-perforator pedicle dangling from undersurface of MSAP free flap allowed reach to recipient site outside zone of injury. (*E*) Early wound healing.

if requisite perforators are absent, access is difficult or obstructed (see **Fig. 7**), or the flap is too thick to allow proper shoe fitting, as is commonly the cause with morbidly obese individuals, then a free flap may be a superior alternative. The donor site of a free flap can be selected from almost anywhere in the body according to the characteristics needed at the recipient site. Reach of a local flap is often constrained by its vascular pedicle, but a free flap should be independent of this restriction. Often the vascular pedicle of a perforator flap actually is too long, creating another enigma to prevent kinking. Whatever the choice, the correct flap selection must be that best to solve the ongoing dilemma in the most expeditious manner.

SUMMARY

In a sense, any revisional foot and ankle surgery causes a disruption of a previously intact skin envelope. In actuality, this then becomes a traumatic injury, with a potential sometimes of serious sequela from deficient wound healing. When that occurs, this acute wound should be approached stepwise similar to the trauma wound; that is, make an accurate assessment of the defect, debride as required, then close by using a suitable modality in a timely fashion.[2] When a vascularized flap is necessary, a team approach, including a reconstructive surgeon familiar with their entire spectrum, would be prudent. The multidisciplinary combination of an orthopedic surgeon and a plastic surgeon has been called the orthoplastic approach to such wounds.[28] If this is instead an issue concerning podiatrists in cooperation with a plastic surgeon, this could appropriately be called a "podiatriplastic" approach.[1] The envisioned goal of all concerned must always be to maximize the lifestyle of the harmed individual by providing the best possible outcome; which, of course, is the ability to ambulate as independently as is possible.[2]

ACKNOWLEDGMENTS

David C. Rice, BS, Physician Extender, Sacred Heart Hospital, Allentown, Pennsylvania, assisted with the operative procedures.

REFERENCES

1. Sinkin JC, Reilly M, Cralley A, et al. Multidisciplinary approach to soft-tissue reconstruction of the diabetic Charcot foot. Plast Reconstr Surg 2015;135:611–6.
2. Hallock GG. The mangled foot and ankle: soft tissue salvage techniques. Clin Podiatr Med Surg 2014;31:565–76.
3. Hollenbeck ST, Woo S, Komatsu I, et al. Longitudinal outcomes and application of the subunit principle to 165 foot and ankle free tissue transfers. Plast Reconstr Surg 2010;125:924–34.
4. Hou Z, Irgit K, Strohecker KA, et al. Delayed flap reconstruction with vacuum-assisted closure management of the open IIIB tibial fracture. J Trauma 2011; 71:1705–8.
5. Kwiecien GJ, Lamaris G, Gharb BB, et al. Long-term outcomes of total knee arthroplasty following soft-tissue defect reconstruction with muscle and fasciocutaneous flaps. Plast Reconstr Surg 2016;137:177e–86e.
6. Hallock GG. The role of free flaps for salvage of the exposed total ankle arthroplasty. Microsurgery 2015;37(1):34–7.
7. Hallock GG. To VAC or not to VAC? Ann Plast Surg 2007;59:473–4.
8. Gottlieb LJ, Krieger LM. From the reconstructive ladder to the reconstructive elevator. Plast Reconstr Surg 1994;93:1503–4.

9. Ullman Y, Fodor L, Ramon Y, et al. The revised reconstructive ladder and its applications for high-energy injuries to the extremities. Ann Plast Surg 2006;56: 401–5.
10. Ghazi BH, Williams JK. Use of integra in complex pediatric wounds. Ann Plast Surg 2011;66:493–6.
11. Park CA, Defranzo AJ, Marks MW, et al. Outpatient reconstruction using integra and subatmospheric pressure. Ann Plast Surg 2009;62:164–9.
12. Hallock GG. Utility of both muscle and fascia flaps in severe lower extremity trauma. J Trauma 2000;48:913–7.
13. Hallock GG. In an era of perforator flaps, are muscle flaps passe? Plast Reconstr Surg 2009;123:1357–63.
14. Hallock GG. If based on citation volume, perforator flaps have landed mainstream. Plast Reconstr Surg 2012;130:769e–71e.
15. Demirtas Y, Ayhan S, Sariguney Y, et al. Distally based lateral and medial leg adipofascial flaps: need for caution with old, diabetic patients. Plast Reconstr Surg 2006;117:272–6.
16. Hallock GG. Foot and ankle reconstruction. In: Blondeel PN, Morris SF, Hallock GG, et al, editors. Perforator flaps: anatomy, technique, and clinical applications, vol. 2, 2nd edition. St Louis (MO): Quality Medical Publishing; 2013. p. 1209–22.
17. Gilbert A. Composite tissue transfers from the foot: anatomic basis and surgical technique. In: Daniller AJ, Strauch B, editors. Symposium on microsurgery. St Louis (MO): CV Mosby; 1976. p. 230–42.
18. Koshima I, Itoh S, Nanba Y, et al. Medial and lateral malleolar perforator flaps for repair of defects around the ankle. Ann Plast Surg 2003;51:579–83.
19. Lu TC, Lin CH, Lin CH, et al. Versatility of the pedicled peroneal artery perforator flaps for soft-tissue coverage of the lower leg and foot defects. J Plast Reconstr Aesth Surg 2011;64:386–93.
20. Hallock GG. Distally based flaps for skin coverage of the foot and ankle. Foot Ankle Int 1996;17:343–8.
21. Behan FC. The keystone design perforator island flap in reconstructive surgery. ANZ J Surg 2003;73:112–20.
22. Hallock GG. The first dorsal metatarsal artery perforator propeller flap. Ann Plast Surg 2016;76:684–7.
23. Jakubietz RG, Jakubietz MG, Gruenert JG, et al. The 180-degree perforator based propeller flap for soft tissue coverage of the distal, lower extremity: a new method to achieve reliable coverage of the distal lower extremity with a local, fasciocutaneous perforator flap. Ann Plast Surg 2007;59:667–71.
24. Liu L, Zou L, Li Z, et al. The extended distally based sural neurocutaneous flap for foot and ankle reconstruction, a retrospective review of 10 years of experience. Ann Plast Surg 2014;72:689–94.
25. Hallock GG. The medial sural medial gastrocnemius perforator free flap: an 'ideal' prone position skin flap. Ann Plast Surg 2004;52:184–7.
26. Hallock GG. Medial sural artery perforator free flap: legitimate use as a solution for the ipsilateral distal lower extremity defect. J Reconstr Microsurg 2014;30: 187–92.
27. Chen SL, Chuang CJ, Chou TD, et al. Free medial sural artery perforator flap for ankle and foot reconstruction. Ann Plast Surg 2005;54:39–43.
28. Lerman OZ, Kovach SJ, Levin LS. The respective roles of plastic and orthopedic surgery in limb salvage. Plast Reconstr Surg 2011;127(Suppl 1):215S–27S.

Current Orthobiologics for Elective Arthrodesis and Nonunions of the Foot and Ankle

George F. Wallace, DPM, MBA

KEYWORDS

• Value analysis • Nonunions • Orthobiologics • Osteoinduction • Osteoconduction

KEY POINTS

- Surgical principles encompassing every facet of an intended procedure need to be followed to increase the probability of fusion.
- Orthobiologics are expensive. Are they absolutely necessary to facilitate an initial fusion or should they be reserved for the nonunion?
- Over the course of time, more and possibly improved orthobiologics will be brought to market in hopes of lessening the nonunion rates of arthrodesis of the foot and ankle. Therefore, foot and ankle surgeons have to be kept informed about these new products.

INTRODUCTION

As in any discussion germane to medicine, there are certain key words and concepts to be initially addressed.

For the broad category of orthobiologics, the important words and definitions used throughout this article and in clinical situations when discussing this topic are defined.

Orthobiologics/Osteobiologics

Orthobiologics/osteobiologics are materials derived to promote formation of bone in arthrodeses, osteotomies, and fractures. They are biologically derived. These terms are for the general heading of a plethora of materials to aid in bone healing.[1] No discussion on the topic is complete without mentioning the seminal work of Urist and colleagues[2,3] in the early 1960s, with the discovery of bone morphogenic protein (BMP) and its function in bone regeneration.

Osteoinduction

In osteoinduction, stem cells are recruited and can be differentiated into osteocytes to aid healing.

The author has nothing to disclose.
Podiatry Service, Ambulatory Care Services, University Hospital, 150 Bergen Street G-142, Newark, NJ 07103, USA
E-mail address: wallacgf@uhnj.org

Osteoconduction

Orthobiologics are inserted as a porous scaffold so bone can proliferate. Additionally they are used as a filler with some use in delayed or nonunions.

Nonunion

Nonunion is the absence of bone healing over 9 months without radiographic evidence of healing over 3 consecutive months. Nonunions never heal on their own. The healing potential has been lost. Delayed unions maintain that potential. Types of nonunions are hypertrophic and atrophic. A general percentage often cited for ankle and rearfoot procedures leading to nonunion is approximately 10%.[4]

Osteogenesis

Osteogenesis provides osteoconductive and osteoinductive properties along with actual fabrication of new bone. Osteoblasts are present within the graft. Only human autograft is osteogenic.

Table 1 lists the types of orthobiologics and provides examples for each.

There are a multitude of products available offering 1 or more of the properties described previously. Their selection depends on whether the application will be during an initial surgery or during a second or even third surgery. Orthobiologics are devised to achieve higher rates of fusion.[1]

SURGICAL PREPARATION

Does the surgeon want to mitigate chances of a nonunion? Then select patients wisely, guarantee compliance, and/or practice sound surgical principles during every case. Even if all of these tenets are followed, however, nonunions can occur. The incidence rate of this complication will never be zero, as would be desired.

Select Patients Wisely

Selecting patients wisely is just about an impossibility. Many patients today have comorbidities and are taking many medicines. A patient who would have been not cleared for surgery years ago is now cleared. Therefore, a thorough medical history is required preoperatively. This alerts the foot and ankle surgeon and begins a discussion of whether an orthobiologic should be used. Some salient findings that may hamper healing are as follows:

- Diabetes especially with neuropathy
- Smoking
- Peripheral artery disease
- Obesity

Table 1
Orthobiologic properties and examples

Osteoinduction	Osteoconduction	Osteogenesis
BMP	Autografts	Autografts
DBM	Allografts	
Allograft chips	DBM	
PRP	Ceramics	
rh-PDGF	Carbon	

Note: Above products will have various trade names.

- Steroid usage
- Collagen disorders
- Osteoporosis/elderly
- Immunosuppression
- Diseases and medications
- Previous surgery in area
- Infection
- High-energy injury
- History of delayed/nonunion[5]

A patient who presents with a displaced trimalleolar ankle fracture needs surgery despite comorbidities that, in a similar patient presenting for hallux abductovalgus surgery, would prohibit that patient from the operating room because of the same medical history.

Guarantee Compliance

Good luck with the concept of patient compliance. How many times are a patient's psyche, social status, communication/understanding of the surgical procedure, and literacy analyzed and are they believed compliant only to see them cut corners and throw compliance out the window? Sometimes it is better to speculate that there is a potential for noncompliance than to be taken by surprise. Fortunately, in the era of value-based medicine, noncompliance has not yet entered the calculation and devalued the foot and ankle surgeon's report card. In the not-too-distant future, noncompliance will be considered and factored in should additional surgeries be required due to a patient's failure to follow instructions (**Fig. 1**).

Sound Surgical Principles

The bone healing cascade cannot be optimized unless surgical principles, including those of AO, are followed. Joint surfaces are prepared. It is the author's preference to resect to cancellous bone rather than at the subchondral bone level. At the former level, however, one has to be cognizant of shortening, hence the possible insertion of a bone graft with orthobiological augmentation if so desired. Where a nonunion exists, the fibrotic and sclerotic tissue is resected completely. A gap is most likely created. A bone graft becomes more likely. Adequate preparation of the joint surfaces then requires stable fixation. Now mix in the above discussions regarding comorbidities and compliance that during the postoperative period signs of healing can be evaluated on the radiographs.

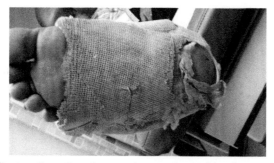

Fig. 1. Noncompliant patient. Cast destroyed yet patient told to be non–weight bearing.

GOLD STANDARD

It can be concluded that the gold standard for any augmentation of bone is an autograft.[4] It is both osteoinductive and osteoconductive. Cortical, cancellous, or a combination bone graft depends on the defect and the type of surgery to be performed. Various donor sites are available, namely the calcaneus, fibula, tibia, and anterior superior iliac crest. Morbidity is associated with each site especially when using the anterior superior iliac crest.[6,7] This most likely needs to be harvested by another surgical specialty.

When another surgeon is used for harvesting of the graft, that physician has to be aware of the amount of bone needed. It is more prudent to procure too much bone than not enough. In one instance, at University Hospital, the surgical team harvesting at the iliac crest was given the dimensions of the graft necessary to fill the defect. Much to the surprise of the author's team performing a talonavicular fusion, the graft procured was too small. In this instance, understanding the amount that had to be procured somehow was lost. Through augmentation with an allograft, the defect was eliminated and the patient went on to complete fusion.

OSTEOINDUCTION MATERIALS

- Autografts
- Bone morphogenic protein (BMP)
  - BMP are growth factors. Due to the quantity of bone needed to harvest BMPs, gene therapy has been used. Currently, 2 recombinant human (rh) BMPs are available: rhBMP-2 and rhBMP-7.[8] There was a concern about a potential cancer risk but a study by Beachler and colleagues[9] has quelled that concern. Fourman and colleagues[10] effectively used BMP with good results in complex ankle arthrodesis.
- Platelet-rich plasma (PRP)
  - PRP was thought to be one of the answers in all types of osseous and musculoskeletal soft tissue injuries. Grant and colleagues[11] used PRP in musculoskeletal injuries and Charcot reconstruction as an augmentation for healing. Of concern is the amount of blood needed and various commercial preparation protocols.[12] These variations in the long run hampers evidence of how much the PRP increases bone healing compared with not using this product. PRP is advocated, however, by Bibbo and Hatfield[13] as an adjunct for bone healing.
- Demineralized Bone Matrix (DBM)
  - DBM is both osteoinductive and osteoconductive. DBM is available in many different forms, from gel to putty to blocks.[8] DBM is the organic component of cortical and cancellous bone after extensive processing.[14] The various processing methods may affect the product in its healing capabilities. DBM's various forms available to the foot and ankle surgeon provide many opportunities for its use in filling bone defects and around grafts. This product is readily available.
- Platelet-derived growth factors (PDGFs)
  - The rh PDGFs are osteoinductive. When combined with a calcium phosphate matrix (tricalcium phosphate [TCP]) it can be used in foot and ankle surgery.[15] Comparison studies are lacking.

OSTEOCONDUCTION MATERIALS

- Autografts
- Allografts

- DBM
- Ceramics—these are synthetic compounds. Commonly used are calcium sulfate, calcium phosphate, and TCP.[16] Composite grafts of calcium sulfate and calcium phosphate are available. Antibiotics may be included in the presence of osteomyelitis. Unlike polymethylmethacrylate, the calcium antibiotic preparation dissolves.
- Carbon may be the future of scaffolding materials. In vitro studies show promise.[17]

ORTHOBIOLOGICS

Within this schema (see **Fig. 5**) are important decision points regarding whether to use orthobiologics. Certain caveats have to be made to guide foot and ankle surgeons:

1. Other than intraoperative findings, surgeons in their preoperative planning should have a good idea whether in general an orthobiologic will be used. Then they should based on the pathology determine if the product should be osteoconductive, osteoinductive, or a combination of both. If not on the shelf, the appropriate product is ordered.
2. What is euphemistically called "redo surgery," comprising nonunions of fractures, malunions, and failed arthrodesis, more than likely requires orthobiologics. Again, the products are chosen based on properties needed to affect union.
3. Unforeseen circumstances intraoperatively always arise; hence, orthobiologics can be considered even in the initial surgical procedure.

VALUE ANALYSIS

As the science for orthobiologics increases and more products are introduced, the cost is probably higher. In an era where hospitals are monitoring costs and reimbursements, using one of the orthobiologics may be barred or limited.

It is incumbent on foot and ankle surgeons to critically analyze any information brought in by sales representatives concerning their products. Clinical and performance questions are asked to foster dialogue. A question regarding the cost of the orthobiologics is never omitted. Surgeons may not be privy to a hospital's reimbursement for a product and surgical case but that should not eliminate the cost question.

Some orthobiologics are in-stock items and easily retrievable during a case. Others, although the representatives would like them to be, in stock have to be brought in on a case-by-case basis until they become, if ever, on the shelf.

Hospitals are loath to allow a product to appear on the doorstep ready to be used without some vetting beforehand. In the perioperative arena, there is usually a go-to person who approves its use on a trial basis.

How can a product get on the shelf?

Different hospitals may use other names, but at University Hospital there is a value analysis committee. Initially a form is completed regarding a product, how/when it is used, its cost, and its complications, if any. The following appear on the committee's New Clinical Request Form:

1. Physician stakeholder (requesting physician)
2. Names of manufacture and sales representative
3. Name of new product or device
4. Type of procedure product used for
5. How will the product improve clinical patient outcomes?
6. Identify evidence-based literature in support of this product outcomes.
7. Anticipated annual volume of use
8. Does the product have Food and Drug Administration approval?

9. Is this new product part of a manufacturer's clinical trial?
10. Is this new product part of an institutional review board research study?
11. How did you become aware of this product?
12. Under conflict of interest:
    a. Have conducted, will conduct, or are conducting research with this product? If yes, funding source?
    b. Is funding pending or have received any?
    c. Employed as a consultant for the manufacturer within the past 2 years?
    d. Current or pending personal investments or other financial interests in this product, manufacturer, or vendor?

Approval can occur more readily if representatives of multiple surgical specialties file applications for the same product. A decision is then made, although after an inordinate amount of time, as to whether a product is approved. Decision support tools are available to facilitate product analysis.[18] Continuous monitoring does occur especially if a product was brought in on great potential only to fizzle out after prolonged use.

Foot and ankle surgeons have to remain vigilant regarding products and report any adverse events. Lifelong learning requires being up to date with the literature, conferences, and opinions gleaned from colleagues.[19] A salesperson should be able to provide literature/studies regarding products and keep surgeons up to date on any future developments (good and bad) regarding the orthobiologic products. Remember there can be an inherent bias with the sales person and their product, however.

CASE 1

A 53-year-old woman presented to the Podiatry Clinic at University Hospital with subtalar arthritis of the right foot along with posterior tibial tendon dysfunction. After the failure of conservative care, a triple arthrodesis was performed (**Fig. 2**).

There are no known allergies. The medical history is unremarkable. No medications are being taken. Examination reveals the following:

1. Vascular status within normal limits
2. Sensation within normal limits
3. Dolor on range of motion of the right subtalar and midtarsal joints without crepitus
4. Radiographs with changes consistent with degenerative joint disease of the right subtalar joint
5. Pes planovalgus right foot with too many toe signs
6. Inability to do double and single heel rises

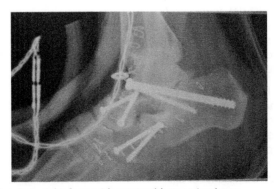

Fig. 2. Triple arthrodesis right foot with external bone stimulator.

A triple arthrodesis along with tendo-Achilles lengthening was performed. No autografts were used or orthobiologics. Fusion was uneventful.

In this particular case, the determination was made not to use adjuncts. Why? The medical history was unremarkable, without any smoking history. Additionally, the joints were never operated on previously. No shortening was anticipated, hence no need for allografts.

This case represents a low risk for a nonunion after the triple arthrodesis. The nonunion rate can be anywhere from 7% to 15%.[8] Could this rate be lowered with the use of orthobiologics? A case of this magnitude is low risk for nonunion and as always becomes a surgeon's preference whether to use orthobiologics.

CASE 2

A 52-year-old woman presented to the Podiatry Clinic at University Hospital with a complaint of a painful, swollen right foot. She acknowledged falling 8 months prior. The foot was "fixed" according to the patient 6 months ago and she would like the hardware removed. Due to an insurance change, the original physician was unable to perform said procedure.

There were no known allergies. The medical history was positive for asthma, anxiety, depression, and obesity. The body mass index was 35. Currently she has smoked 2 cigarettes per day for the past 38 years. Medications are aripiprazole, alprazolam, zolpidem, and albuterol.

Examination reveals the following:

1. Vascular status within normal limits
2. Sensation within normal limits
3. Medial and lateral fine-lined cicatrices
4. Pain along the scars when palpated but no Tinel sign evident
5. Dolor on range of motion of right subtalar and midtarsal joints with no crepitus. The ranges of motion were restricted, however.
6. Radiographs (**Fig. 3**) depict attempted right triple arthrodesis with nonunions of the subtalar, talonavicular, and calcaneocuboid articulations.
7. Pes planovalgus bilateral with semirigid forefoot varus on the right side

Subsequently, under general anesthesia after hardware removal and tendo-Achilles lengthening, the nonunions were addressed. Each joint surface was débrided to raw bleeding bone. Appropriate-sized allografts were inserted in the 3 joints. A commercial product consisting of B-TCP (granules) and rhPDGF was used in all of the joints to be fused. A posterior splint was applied and the patient instructed to remain non–weight bearing (**Fig. 4**).

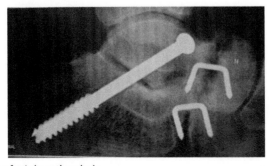

Fig. 3. Nonunion of triple arthrodesis.

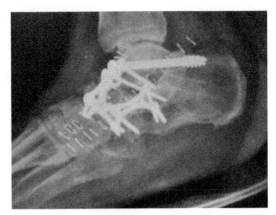

Fig. 4. Triple arthrodesis using allograft and a B-TCP and rhPDGF product.

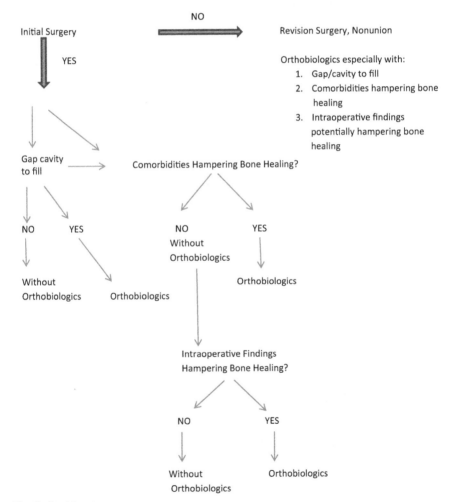

Fig. 5. Decision tree.

How was the decision made to use both the allograft and proprietary material?

Resection of the fibrotic tissue constituting the nonunion to bleeding bone left large deficits in each joint. Therefore, allografts were inserted.

The fusion sites were augmented, with the orthobiologic to facilitate union. In any redo surgery, it is in the best interest of the patient to optimize as much as possible the potential to heal the fusion sites. It could be postulized that the fusion of the initial surgery did not occur due to fixation malposition and subsequent failure. Not knowing the actual preparation technique and compliance, however, the foot and ankle surgeon has to almost throw the kitchen sink at the problem. An external bone stimulator was used also in keeping with this analogy.

Note the thought process in Case 2 versus Case 1, where the fusion was a first-time event and not performed at another institution by another unknown surgeon (**Fig. 5**).

The risk of a nonunion in this case can be considered high due to the previous surgical intervention and nonunion already in place. Orthobiologics become an added boost to facilitate healing.

The material was brought in for this 1-time use. An application was submitted to the value analysis committee for continued use of this product.

SUMMARY/QUESTIONS

There are pertinent thought-provoking summary points/questions to be made:

1. The evidence for use of the products discussed is not robust, especially in the foot and ankle literature.[20] Outcome data need to be more rigorous, especially to compare the fusion rates of one product to another and to controls. Manufacturer preparation for the various products hampers adequate conclusions.
2. Cost in this era of concern can play into whether to use a product or whether it is available in a surgeon's operating room. Value analysis becomes a conduit to bringing a product on board.
3. Are the various products used in all initial surgeries or in those that are being redone? Patient history plays a large role.
4. The overall nonunion rate is cited at 10% for ankle and rearfoot surgeries. Can it ever be zero? What would be a good reduction of that 10% rate using these products?
5. Can the various products be compared even in the same class when proprietary manufacturing may differ from product to product?
6. What is the next product? How does the foot and ankle surgeon analyze this product or is it just by trial and error?
7. Are orthobiologies to be used in every surgery?
8. Readers are urged to reread the articles cited in this issue. If and when would an orthobiologic product be used and which one?

REFERENCES

1. Egol KA, Nauth A, Lee M, et al. Bone grafting: sourcing, timing, strategies, and alternatives. J Orthop Trauma 2015;29(12):S10–4.
2. Urist MR. Bone: formation by autoinduction. Science 1965;150:893–9.
3. Urist MR, Silverman BF, Buring K, et al. The bone induction principle. Clin Orthop 1967;53:243–83.
4. Arner JW, Santrock RD. A historical review of common bone graft materials in foot and ankle surgery. Foot Ankle Spec 2014;7(2):143–51.
5. Bibbo C, Nelson J, Ehrlich BR. Bone morphogenetic proteins: indications and uses. Clin Podiatr Med Surg 2015;32(1):35–43.

6. Roberts TT, Rosenbaum AJ. Bone grafts, bone substitutes and orthobiologics. Organogenesis 2012;8(4):114–24.

7. Derner R, Anderson AC. The bone morphogenic protein. Clin Podiatr Med Surg 2005;22(4):607–18.

8. Malay DS, Harris W. Orthobiologics. In: Sutherland JT, editor. McGlamry's comprehensive textbook of foot and ankle surgery. 4th edition. Philadelphia: Wolters Kluwer Health; 2013. p. 1322–32.

9. Beachler DC, Yanik EL, Martin BI, et al. Bone morphogenetic protein use and cancer risk among patients undergoing lumbar arthrodesis. J Bone Joint Surg Am 2016;98(13):1064–72.

10. Fourman MS, Borst EW, Bogner E, et al. Recombinant human BMP-2 increases the incidence and rate of healing in complex ankle arthrodesis. Clin Orthop Relat Res 2014;472:732–9.

11. Grant WP, Jerlin EA, Pietrzak WS, et al. The utilization of autologous growth factors for the facilitation of fusion in complex neuropathic fractures in the diabetic population. Clin Podiatr Med Surg 2005;22(4):561–84.

12. Malhotra A, Pelletier MH, Yu Y, et al. Can platelet-rich plasma (PRP) improve bone healing? A comparison between the theory and experimental outcomes. Arch Orthop Trauma Surg 2013;133(2):153–65.

13. Bibbo C, Hatfield PS. Platelet-rich plasma concentrate to augment bone fusion. Foot Ankle Clin 2010;15(4):641–9.

14. Stern SF, Pacaccio DJ. Demineralized bone matrix: basic science and clinical applications. Clin Podiatr Med Surg 2005;22(4):599–606.

15. DiGiovanni CW, Lin SS, Baumhauer JF, et al. Recombinant human platelet-derived growth factor- BB and beta- tricalcium phosphate (rh PDGF- BB/B-TCP): an alternative to autogenous bone graft. J Bone Joint Surg Am 2013; 95(13):1184–92.

16. Panchbhavi VK. Synthetic bone grafting in foot and ankle surgery. Foot Ankle Clin 2010;15(4):559–76.

17. Czarnecki JS, Lafdi K, Tonis PA. The future of carbon-based scaffolds in foot and ankle surgery. Clin Podiatr Med Surg 2015;32(1):73–91.

18. Martelli N, Hansen P, Vanden Brink H, et al. Combining multi-criteria decision analysis and mini-health technology assessment: a funding decision support tool for medical devices in a university hospital setting. J Biomed Inform 2016; 59:201–8.

19. Raza R, Commarasamy A, Khan KS. Best evidence continuous medical education. Arch Gynecol Obstet 2009;280(4):683–7.

20. Lin SS, Yeranosian MG. What's new in foot and ankle surgery. J Bone Joint Surg Am 2016;98(10):874–80.

Index

Note: Page numbers of article titles are in **boldface** type.

Clin Podiatr Med Surg 34 (2017) 409–413
http://dx.doi.org/10.1016/S0891-8422(17)30046-0
0891-8422/17

podiatric.theclinics.com

Moving?

Make sure your subscription moves with you!

To notify us of your new address, find your **Clinics Account Number** (located on your mailing label above your name), and contact customer service at:

Email: journalscustomerservice-usa@elsevier.com

800-654-2452 (subscribers in the U.S. & Canada)
314-447-8871 (subscribers outside of the U.S. & Canada)

Fax number: 314-447-8029

Elsevier Health Sciences Division
Subscription Customer Service
3251 Riverport Lane
Maryland Heights, MO 63043

*To ensure uninterrupted delivery of your subscription, please notify us at least 4 weeks in advance of move.

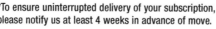